D1082861

Ex-Library: Friends of
Lake County Public Library

The Elephant Man

Other books
by Ashley Montagu...

Man's Most Dangerous Myth:
    The Fallacy of Race
The Humanization of Man
Man in Process
Human Heredity
The Cultured Man
Man: His First Two Million Years
Coming into Being Among
    the Australian Aborigines
Edward Tyson, M.D., F.R.S. (1650-1708)
    and the Rise of Human and
    Comparative Anatomy in England
Statement on Race
The Direction of Human Development
The Natural Superiority of Women
The Reproductive Development
    of the Female
On Being Human
The Biosocial Nature of Man
Darwin, Competition and Cooperation
On Being Intelligent
Immortality, Religion, and Morals
Education and Human Relations
Anthropology and Human Nature
Introduction to Physical Anthropology
Handbook of Anthropometry
Prenatal Influences
Race, Science, and Humanity
Life Before Birth
The Science of Man
Anatomy and Physiology,
    2 vols. (with E. Steen)
The Nature of Human Aggression
Sex, Man and Society
Man Observed
The Human Revolution
The Idea of Race
Up the Ivy
Growing Young
Touching: The Human Significance
    of the Skin
The American Way of Life

The Anatomy of Swearing
The Peace of the World
The Prevalence of Nonsense
    (with E. Darling)
The Ignorance of Certainty
    (with E: Darling)
Human Evolution (with C. L. Brace)
Textbook of Human Genetics
    (with M. Levitan)
The Dolphin in History (with John Lilly)
Man and the Computer
    (with S. S. Snyder)
The Human Connection
    (with Floyd W. Matson)
The Dehumanization of Man
    (with Floyd W. Matson)

Editor

Studies and Essays in the History
    of Science and Learning
Toynbee and History
The Meaning of Love
Genetic Mechanisms in Human Disease
International Pictorial Treasury
    of Knowledge
Atlas of Human Anatomy
Culture and the Evolution of Man
Culture: Man's Adaptive Dimension
The Concept of Race
The Concept of the Primitive
Man and Aggression
The Human Dialogue
    (with F. E. Matson)
Readings on the Origin
    and Evolution of Man
Race & IQ
Learning Non-Aggression
Culture and Human Development
The Practice of Love
Frontiers of Anthropology
The Endangered Environment
Sociobiology Examined
Science, Evolution and Creationism
Marriage: Past and Present

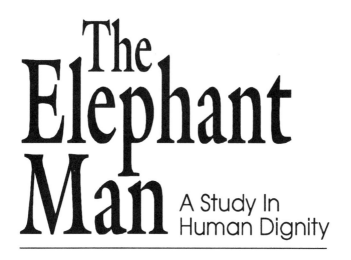

The Elephant Man

A Study In
Human Dignity

ASHLEY   MONTAGU

LAKE COUNTY PUBLIC LIBRARY

Acadian House
PUBLISHING
LAFAYETTE, LOUISIANA

ABOUT THE COVER: Joseph Merrick, "the Elephant Man," puts the finishing touches on one of the cardboard models he made while living in the London Hospital. For a number of years the hospital was his home, his shelter from the cold, cruel world of his previous existence as a curiosity in traveling freak shows.

3 3113 01953 1435

Copyright © 1971, 1979, 1996 by Ashley Montagu

All rights reserved, including the right to reproduce this book or portions thereof in any form whatsoever. For information, contact Acadian House Publishing, P.O. Box 52247, Lafayette, Louisiana 70505.

Library of Congress Catalog Card Number: 95-79903

ISBN: 0-925417-17-3

Third Edition

♦ **Published by Acadian House Publishing, Lafayette, Louisiana (Edited by Trent Angers; graphic design by Tom Sommers)**

♦ **Cover illustration by Patrick Soper, Lafayette, Louisiana**

♦ **Color separation by Grand Masters Colour, Portland, Oregon**

♦ **Printed by BookCrafters, Fredericksburg, Virginia**

Preface

It was shortly after its publication, in 1923, that I first read Frederick Treves' *The Elephant Man and Other Reminiscences.* I was immediately fascinated by the title-story.

"The Elephant Man" story held a special appeal for me, for I was at that time a student of that unlikely combination of subjects, human anatomy and behavior. In addition to the title-story, Treves' other reminiscences circumnavigated an institution, the London Hospital, which as a boy I had known both intra- and extra-murally for many years. I was thoroughly familiar with the *mise en scène* and, indeed, with almost every place of which Treves wrote.

His book dealt with events which had occurred not long before I was born, in a district of London which has always had a strange romantic appeal, and to which the distance of time has added a peculiar enchantment.

For me, then, the writing of this book had a threefold appeal: human nature, anatomy, and the London of Henry Mayhew. The book is the result of that combination of interests.

It is, first, about two extraordinary men – one a "freak" of nature named Joseph Merrick, the Elephant Man, the other a distinguished surgeon and teacher, Frederick Treves – and a loving mother whose care and nurturing play a critical role in the unfolding of our story. Second, it is about the development of human behavior. And, third, it is about the nature of the astonishing disorder from which the Elephant Man suffered. But, I suppose, what the book is finally really about is love and the triumph of the human spirit over adversity.

Since the First and Second Editions of the book were published, in 1971 and 1979, respectively, further research in England and elsewhere has enabled me to throw some new light on the early history of Joseph Merrick, as well as to render some matters clearer than they were before. These additions and corrections are incorporated into this Third Edition of *The Elephant Man.*

In this edition I have corrected a number of errors which were mainly due to the fact that I relied largely upon Sir Frederick Treves' account of The Elephant Man. Even in the absence of any other knowledge of Joseph Merrick – whom for some strange reason Treves miscalled "John" – I could not accept much that Treves had to say, particularly about the relationship between Merrick and his mother. In the light of what we have learned about the human psyche down through the years, it was clear to me that Treves must have gotten an essential part of our hero's history wrong.

It was, therefore, gratifying to me to find my views confirmed in Michael Howell and Peter Ford's book, *The True History of the Elephant Man*, published in 1980. That book has made it possible to clear up some mysteries that obscured Merrick's history.

In addition to the revision of the text the present edition has enabled me to add some new illustrations, and in some cases to improve upon the old.

Finally, what is most gratifying is that as a result of the publicity Joseph Merrick's story has received – the books and articles, the plays, the movie, the TV specials – an organization has been formed dedicated to the encouragement, support, and dissemination of information relating to the disorder from which Merrick suffered. That organization is The National Neurofibromatosis Foundation, Inc., (141 Fifth Avenue, New York, N.Y. 10010.) There are today chapters in every state of the country.

The research the Foundation and its chapters have supported, made possible by voluntary contributions from the public, has led to the spectacular discovery of the genes responsible for neurofibromatosis. These discoveries constitute a tribute to the spirit of "the Elephant Man." These discoveries will undoubtedly lead eventually to the prevention of the development of neurofibromatosis and its side effects. Joseph Merrick would have rejoiced to know that so much good could have come from the story of his heroic life.

–Ashley Montagu
27 July 1995   Princeton, New Jersey

Dedicated to the Memory
of
Charles S. Sonntag
Demonstrator in Human Anatomy
at
University College, London, 1922-1925

Acknowledgements

In the course of my study of the Elephant Man I have been most generously aided by Professor Richard J. Harrison, formerly Professor of Anatomy at the London Hospital Medical College, and later Professor of Anatomy at the University of Cambridge. I owe an especial debt of gratitude to him for his many courtesies, beginning as long ago as 1950.

I am also much indebted to the authorities at the London Hospital Medical College for their permission to examine the skeleton and casts of The Elephant Man, and for the pains they took in making most of the photographs for me which illustrate this volume. To Mr. E. P. Entract, Librarian to the London Hospital Medical College, I owe thanks for the photographs of the Hospital and the College. To the American Medical Association and Dr. Lawrence M. Solomon I am obliged for permission to reprint his essay on "Quasimodo's Diagnosis" as Appendix 3.

For permission to reprint the title-story from *The Elephant Man and Other Reminiscences*, I am obliged to Messrs. Cassell & Co., Ltd. of London.

I am most grateful to the Librarians of the College of Physicians of Philadelphia, and of Princeton University, for their many kind offices.

For supplying some of the illustrations for this Third Edition, and for much other assistance, I am indebted to Mr. P. G. Nunn, Assistant Curator, Museum Department, London Hospital Medical College. I am grateful also to Mr. Nicholas Reed for sending me a copy of his article on the mystery of Treves' misadventure with Joseph Merrick's given name, as well as a copy of the original manuscript of Treves' essay on the Elephant Man. Finally, I am much indebted to Trent Angers, the publisher of the Third Edition, for his devotion to the welfare of this book.

– A.M.

x

Contents

The Elephant Man

Chapter One

Discovering 'The Elephant Man'

Life, like a dome of many-coloured glass,
Stains the white radiance of Eternity,
Until Death tramples it to fragments.
  —Shelley, *Adonais*

What is a human life? A pulse in the heartbeat of eternity? A cry that begins with birth and ends with death? A brief and tempestuous sojourn on an inhospitable shore, where there is really neither joy, nor love, nor light, nor certitude, nor peace, nor help for pain?

Or is it, is it, something more?

In this book, I think, lies something of the answer to these questions. It is a true story. It happened in the eighties of the past century. It is from many angles of vision an enthralling and ennobling story.

It tells us something not only about the darker but also about the brighter sides of human nature, of the spontaneous kindness to which human beings are disposed, as well as the unfeeling cruelty of which others are capable, but above all else of the supreme human integrity which some members of the species *Homo sapiens* are able to maintain in the face of never-ending adversities of the most devastating kinds.

The central hero of this story, "the Elephant Man," whose name was Joseph Merrick, lived just short of 28 years, most of

1

them spent in a living purgatory. Hideously deformed, malodorous, for the most part maltreated, constantly in pain, lame, fed the merest scraps, exhibited as a grotesque monster at circuses, fairs, and wherever else a penny might be turned, the object of constant expressions of horror and disgust, it might have been expected that "the Elephant Man" would have grown into a creature detesting all human beings, bitter, awkward, difficult in his relations with others, ungentle, unfeeling, aggressive, and unlovable.

But such was not the case. And it is this that makes his story, tragic as it is, so doubly fascinating and heartening.

From the day I first heard of the story of "the Elephant Man," in 1923, I was fascinated and eager to find out more. At the time, I was a student attending University College in London, studying human nature, anthropology and the biological social sciences.

The story was originally brought to the attention of English readers by Sir Frederick Treves, the leading English surgeon of his day, in his book, *The Elephant Man and Other Reminiscences.* Treves had intended to write his reminiscences about his famous patients, but changed his mind and wrote instead of his unknown patients, of whom "the Elephant Man" was undoubtedly the most remarkable.

His book was published in February 1923 and was reprinted in the same month, then again in October, once more in May 1924, and again in June 1928. A paperback edition was issued in 1941. In all its editions the book has become a great rarity.

I borrowed the book from a bookshop and read it in October 1923. The first of the book's 12 chapters, in which Treves gives an account of "the Elephant Man," is the most dramatic and the most moving. It made the deepest impression on me. In the course of my years as an anatomist, anthropologist, and teacher of medical students and would-be psychiatrists and neurologists, I often had occasion to recall "the Elephant Man" and to tell his story.

From about 1940 onward I attempted in vain to secure a copy

of Treves' book. Then, by happy chance, a friend of mine who knew of my interest in the book came upon a copy of the paperback edition in Cairo and sent it to me. To this day it is the only copy I have seen since 1923. None of the booksellers' catalogues in which I have hunted through the years has ever listed a copy.

For some 30 years I intermittently endeavored to interest various publishers in the book I wanted to write on "the Elephant Man" and his rescuers but without success. The book might never have been published had not my friend and anthropological colleague Edmund Carpenter told David Outerbridge, who had just then commenced publishing in New York, that I had a story to tell that no one wanted to publish. David came out to Princeton to see me. I told him the story and the book I wished to write about it, and showed him the photographs and other materials relating to "the Elephant Man." He was interested and agreed to publish the book. The first edition came out in 1971; the second in 1979.

I had long harbored the hope that the book – if I could ever get a publisher to see the value of it – would rescue "the Elephant Man" and his benefactor from the oblivion into which they had fallen. That hope was satisfied beyond my expectations. Not only was the book well received in the United States, Canada and England, but it also excited the interests of many talented people who went on to create dramatic works of art based on "the Elephant Man's" story. At least half a dozen movie scripts were written, a movie was made, eight or ten plays were written, seven of which were produced and performed in the U.S., England and France, and a bevy of books, essays, poems and feature articles were written and distributed. As an article in the 7 March 1979 edition of *Variety* Magazine put it:

"A herd of 'Elephant Men' is proliferating on U.S. stages."

What was it in the story of "the Elephant Man" that struck such a chord not only with the writers, poets and producers but also in the minds and hearts of the readers and viewers? Was it their sense of empathy and compassion for the plight of "the Elephant Man?" Was it their admiration for the British surgeon who rescued him from the miserable circumstances of his life? Or was it that they were, perhaps, in search of some element of truth, some moral, that would help them to close the gap between the kind of human beings they were and the kind of human beings they longed to become?

In a very real sense, this is the story not only of Joseph Merrick, "the Elephant Man," but also of Frederick Treves, the British surgeon who liberated and befriended him, and Mary Jane Merrick, the loving mother who reared and nurtured him for the long and painful journey which lay ahead.

Before we proceed with our inquiry into this heroic journey into the night, the story itself must be told and the first of our main characters introduced.

Chapter Two

Frederick Treves

*F*rederick Treves came of old yeomen stock native to Dorset for centuries. He was born in Dorchester, Dorset, 15 February 1853, the youngest son of William Treves, a well-to-do furniture dealer and upholsterer, and his wife Jane, daughter of John Knight of Honiton, some 30 miles northwest of Dorchester.

At the age of seven Frederick Treves was sent to the school kept by the Dorset poet, the Reverend William Barnes (1801-1886). Here he remained for two years. Barnes, who had commenced schoolmastering in 1822 after obtaining his degree from Cambridge, was a man of extraordinary genius. Among his many accomplishments were those of engraver, musician, naturalist, linguist, philologist, humanist, educator and poet. His bucolic, often very moving, poems, published in a series of three volumes, *Poems of Rural Life in the Dorset Dialect,* between the years 1844 and 1862, had made him well known to the reading public, but were scarcely rewarded enough to free him from the poverty and financial worries which haunted him during the greater part of his life.

As an educator Barnes was many years ahead of his time, teaching with love and affection. His chief means of instruction consisted of discourses delivered as he walked up and down the room. His favorite subjects were logic and grammar, and on Treves' first day at school the subject was, "Logic is the Art of the Right Use of Reason." Quite mystifying to a boy of seven, but unforgettable. Treves to the end of his life carried with him the singular little pocket grammar that Barnes published for the benefit of his class.

It has been said that the greatest gift a teacher can make to his students is his own personality. In this Barnes seems to have richly succeeded with the impressionable young Treves, as he did with many other students. Treves never forgot the qualities of kindness and understanding of his teacher, and in his own relations with students and patients in later life he never failed to exhibit the same traits. In his book *Highways and Byeways of Dorset* (London: Macmillan & Co., 1906) and in his essay "William Barnes, the Dorset Poet" (London: *The Dorset Yearbook, 1915-1916)* Treves wrote of his years at school with love and admiration for his old schoolmaster, "a genius whom few recognized." It is evident that Treves' love of literature and his fondness for words were first aroused and developed under the charismatic influence of Barnes.

In his youth Treves was an athlete, a great swimmer who loved the water, subsequently becoming a master of sailing and a qualified mariner.

In 1864, at the age of 11, Treves entered Merchant Taylors School in London. Following the completion of his studies there he entered University College, University of London, and in 1871, at the age of 18, he entered upon the study of medicine at the London Hospital. In 1874 he passed the examinations for the Licensure of Apothecaries Hall, and in the following year he successfully completed the examinations for the Membership of the Royal College of Surgeons. In the same year, 1875, he became house-surgeon at the London Hospital, and in 1876 he took up a post as resident medical officer at the Royal National Hospital for Scrofula at Margate, on the south coast, a hospital to which his elder brother William, his senior by ten years, was honorary surgeon.

In 1877, at the age of 24, Treves married Anne Elizabeth, youngest daughter of a Dorchester merchant, Alfred Samuel Mason, and went into practice at Wirksworth, Derbyshire. In the following year Treves took the Fellowship of the Royal College of Surgeons. In 1879 he gave up general practice to assume the surgical registrarship at the London Hospital. He was appointed assistant-surgeon in the same year, and became full consulting surgeon in 1884. (This was the year he was to meet "the Elephant Man" for the first time.) He was also appointed a demonstrator in anatomy at the London Hospital Medical College, and was in charge of the practical teaching of anatomy from 1881 to 1884, when he became lecturer, a post he held until 1893. In the latter year he resigned the lectureship in anatomy to become lecturer in surgery, a post in which he continued until 1897.[1]

In 1883 Treves published what became the most widely read work of its kind, his *Surgical Applied Anatomy*. In 1901 Treves, no longer having the necessary time, enlisted the collaboration of Arthur Keith, who was then teaching anatomy at the London Hospital Medical College, in revising the book, a task in which Keith was involved until 1914, when he turned over the work to another anatomist. The work flourished for more than half a century and served students and surgeons all over the world as the best and most authoritative work on the subject.

In 1885, enlarging upon an interest he had developed earlier, Treves published a small book on the *Influence of Clothing Upon Health* in which he discussed the many undesirable features of women's clothing, such as corsetting and tight lacing, including much that was anticipatory of the changes that have come about in women's clothing.

In the Medical College Treves soon established himself as an outstanding personality. An excellent teacher and surgical operator, he was very popular with the students, and was elected the first president of the Students' Union, an organization which he helped to found. Keith, who in later years was my teacher, knew Treves well for some 30 years. He spoke of him as a man of nimble wit, good-natured and cheerful, a good companion, and renowned for his ability to tell a story well, but who left no permanent mark in the field of surgery.[2] This latter observation is incomprehensible, for Treves' work on the treatment of intestinal obstruction and his advocacy of early operation in appendicitis would alone be sufficient to count as a "permanent mark."

Of Treves' style Keith wrote: "He knew how to give the dull facts of anatomy a picturesque setting; he was a master of emphatic phrase; as a demonstrator of anatomy he had learned the art of attracting the wandering attention of the medical student by the use of apt similies."

During the '80s Treves' surgical practice grew apace. His office at 6 Wimpole St. became one of the best known in England. In 1898, at the age of 45, Treves resigned his lectureship at the hospital to devote full time to his increasingly lucrative practice. (At his death, 25 years later, Treves left an estate valued at more than £100,000.)

Treves' patients were mainly drawn from the wealthy, high society, the nobility, and the Royal Family. His rooms at Wimpole Street were so crowded that he customarily put his patients in every available room in the house while they were waiting to be seen by him. Lady Treves used to say that the only room she had to herself was her bedroom. Treves received the hundred-guinea fee, then the upper limit for a surgeon, more often than any other surgeon of his day. But even as the leading and busiest surgeon of his time, Treves never forgot his poor patients. On Sundays, his only free day, he regularly attended the hospital to examine the cases in his wards more thoroughly and at greater leisure than was possible during weekdays when students and visitors required much of his attention at the bedside. Following the completion of his rounds he would take a 40- or 50-mile bicycle ride.

In 1900 Treves was appointed Surgeon-Extraordinary to Queen Victoria. He also became Surgeon-in-Ordinary to the Duke of York, and later Sergeant Surgeon to King George V, and Surgeon-in-Ordinary to Queen Alexandra. He was made a Commander of the Bath, and in 1901 Knight Commander of the Victorian Order. During all this time Treves was busily engaged in producing books and monographs on surgical anatomy, operative procedures and intestinal disorders.

It was, therefore, natural that, when just before his coronation in January 1902, King Edward VII fell gravely ill with a painful intestinal disorder, Treves should have been called in. Treves confirmed the diagnosis as acute appendicitis, a condition upon which he was the leading surgical authority. Treves advised immediate operation. To this, the King, who was both alarmed and obdurate, demurred. He was determined to proceed with his coronation on the 26th of January rather than disappoint the nation.

"In that case, Sir," Treves is reported to have said, "you will go to the Abbey as a corpse."

After a scene of prolonged and painful pleading the King was ultimately persuaded. A room was specially prepared in Buckingham Palace for the operation, and the next morning King Edward, conducted by his wife, Queen Alexandra, entered the room, lay down on the operating table, and was promptly put under an anesthetic. The King began to throw his arms about and grow black in the face, while the Queen struggled to hold him down, crying out, "Why don't you begin?"

To his consternation Treves realized that the Queen intended to remain in the room throughout the operation. Treves wrote later:

"I was anxious to prepare for the operation, but did not like to take off my coat, tuck up my sleeves, and put on an apron while the Queen was present." [3]

Treves gently but firmly told the Queen she must leave, which, bowing to superior authority, she reluctantly agreed to do. Forty minutes later Treves emerged to tell her that the operation had been a complete success. It was the day on which the King was to have been crowned. For the second time in his life King Edward had been at death's door and had survived.

That year Treves was made a Baronet and promoted to

Grand Commander of the Victorian Order.

In 1906 Treves was elected Lord Rector of the University of Aberdeen. This honor required no more than a single address on the appointed day. Treves happily accepted the invitation, but on condition that the traditional student interruptions be omitted. On the occasion of the Rectorial Address it was the tradition among students to punctuate the oration with appropriate expressions of approval or disapproval by handclapping, foot-stomping, and more vocal forms of commentary. Treves delivered his lecture, and so great was the respect in which he was held by the students that there was, in fact, not a single interruption during the whole hour of his address.

Treves held that after 55 no surgeon should operate, and so at that age he retired, in 1908, from the active practice of surgery to live in Thatched House Lodge in Richmond Park. This house was lent him by King Edward, with whom he remained on terms of close and confidential friendship, a friendship that was continued with his son, King George V. In the following years Treves and his wife traveled widely, in the West Indies, Palestine, Uganda, and many other places. These travels led to a series of books.

Lady Treves said that her husband was never happier than when he had a pen in his hand. The truth is that his real love was literature. This is very evident from his various writings. Even his technical works were elegantly written.

After the 1914-18 war, during which Treves had served as President of the Headquarters Medical Board at the War Office, and was actively engaged in the work of the International Red Cross, sudden heart attacks began to afflict him. Continuing failing health compelled him to move abroad in 1920, first to Evian on the Savoy side of Lake Geneva. It was here that Treves wrote *The Riviera of the Corniche Road* (1921), *The Lake Geneva* (1922), and his last book, *The Elephant Man and Other Reminiscences* (1923).

In 1922 Treves suffered a severe attack of pneumonia, from which he seemed to recover. *The Elephant Man* appeared at the beginning of February 1923 and was widely and well reviewed. In the autumn of the same year Treves moved into an apartment

at Vevey on the Swiss side of Lake Geneva. There he was taken
ill on the 3rd of December with peritonitis. He was quickly
removed to a nursing home in Lausanne, but it was too late to
do anything for him, and on 7 December 1923 he died. His body
was cremated, and on 2 January 1924 his ashes were brought to
Dorchester Cemetery, where, after a brief ceremony at which
his old friend Thomas Hardy was present, what remained of
Frederick Treves was buried. The event was commemorated by
Hardy in a poem, "In The Evening."

In The Evening
In Memoriam Frederick Treves, 1853-1923
(Dorchester Cemetery, Jan. 2, 1924)

In the evening, when the world knew he was dead,
    He lay amid the dust and hoar
Of ages; and to a spirit attending said:
      "This chalky bed?–
I surely seem to have been here before?"

"O yes. You have been here. You knew the place,
    Substanced as you, long ere your call;
And if you cared to do so you might trace
      In this gray space
Your being, and the being of men all."

Thereto said he: "Then why was I called away?
    I knew no trouble or discontent:
Why did I not prolong my ancient stay
      Herein for aye?"
The spirit shook its head. "None knows: you went.

"And though, perhaps, Time did not sign to you
    The need to go, dream-vision sees
How Aesculapius' phantom hither flew,
      With Galen's, too,
And his of Cos – plague-proof Hippocrates,

"And beckoned you forth, whose skill had read as theirs,
    Maybe, had Science chanced to spell
In their day, modern modes to stem despairs
      That mankind bears! . . .
Enough. You have returned. And all is well."

Treves had two daughters, the younger of whom pre-deceased him, dying tragically following an operation for the very disease on which Treves was the world's leading surgical authority, acute appendicitis. Dying without male issue, the baronetcy that had been conferred on Treves lapsed and became extinct.

Chapter Three

Downtown London, 1884

*A*t the time of his discovery of the Elephant Man in November of 1884, Treves was 31 years of age, a surgeon at the London Hospital and lecturer in anatomy at the London Hospital Medical College.

The London Hospital was the largest institution of its kind in the British Empire, occupying a site of many acres in the middle of the poverty-stricken center of the East End of London. The hospital is situated on Whitechapel Road, a wide and commodious thoroughfare built by the Romans.

The London Hospital was founded in 1740 and its main building was erected in 1759. The principal buildings are situated on the south side of Whitechapel Road. The London Hospital Medical College, which enjoys the distinction of being the first medical college to be established in association with a hospital upon the model of the faculty of a university, stands on the west side of the main building, opposite the large Church of St. Philip, which will figure in our story later.

Because of its situation in the midst of the slums of London, in "the roughest and most unsavory part of the town," as

Treves himself described it, its more than eight hundred beds, its enormous number of inpatients and still greater number of outpatients, "The London," as it came to be called, had a great appeal for aspiring students of medicine and medical men of every description. Here could be seen every possible kind of disease and disorder. The experience one could gain at "The London" could scarcely be equalled anywhere else in the world.[4] It was the knowledge of this fact that probably brought the young Frederick Treves to the London Hospital.

On both the north and south sides of Whitechapel Road the pavements, like the cobbled road, are unusually ample, and give support to innumerable small shops. In spite of the bombings of two World Wars, fires, demolitions, rebuilding, and the replacement of horse-drawn vehicles by motor-driven traffic, the appearance of the area remains little changed from what it was in Treves' days at "The London."

During weekdays, and especially on Saturdays, the north side of the road affords on its spacious pavements accommodation for the most colorful of markets. Movable wheelbarrows and stalls by the dozen offer everything for sale from apples and secondhand books to zithers and zippers. From early times the broad expanse of Whitechapel Road also had served as a hay market, but with the increase and hazards of motor traffic the hay market was finally discontinued in 1928.

A feel for the atmosphere of the Whitechapel market in Treves' day – and for what life was like for the poor and abandoned of London – can be gotten from the observations of Blanchard Jerrold in his book, *London: A Pilgrimage,* published in 1872:

> It is an ancient neighbourhood, as some of the overhanging houses proclaim; and it remains a picturesque one, with the infinitely various lines and contrivances of the shops and stalls, and gaudy inns and public houses; the overhanging clothes, the mounds of vegetables, the piles of hardware, the confused heaps of fish, all cast about to catch the pence of the bonnetless dishevelled

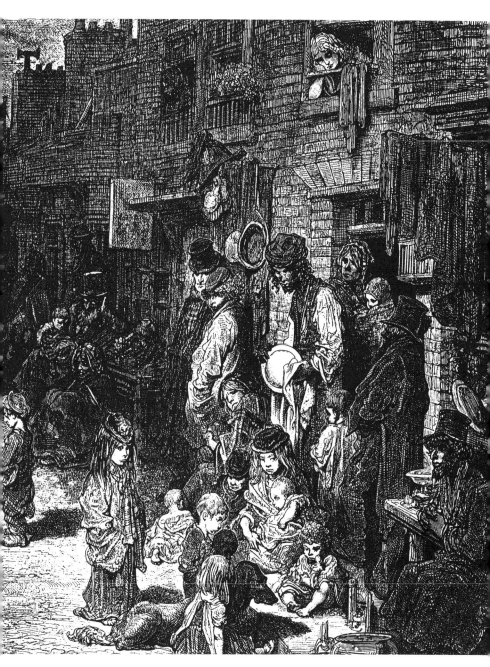

Figure 1. The Elephant Man was first seen by Frederick Treves in a neighborhood such as this in downtown London in November of 1884. (Illustration by Gustave Doré from *London: A Pilgrimage*, published in 1872.)

women, the heavy navvies, and the shoeless children. The German, the Jew, the Frenchman, the Lascar, the swarthy native of Spitalfields, the leering thin-handed thief, the bully of his court, the silly-Billy of the neighbourhood – on whom the neighbourhood is merciless – with endless swarms of ragged children, fill road and pavement.

In Treves' day Whitechapel Road presented a rather more squalid appearance than it does today. The small, neglected shops were a great deal more dingy, and lit by gaslight were dismally uninviting. The poor and abandoned were very much more in evidence, and owing to the poverty of the people, shopkeepers, eking out a precarious living, tended to go out of business with discouraging regularity. The empty shops would stand unrented for months, sometimes years, padlocked, shuttered, dirty, and decaying. Signs in shop windows reading "This Shop to Let" were a common sight. Sometimes a shop would be rented for a short time by a wandering gypsy fortune-teller or an itinerant showman, and as quickly be vacated again.

It was in one such vacant shop on an afternoon late in November of 1884 that Frederick Treves first came upon the Elephant Man.

Chapter Four

The Elephant Man

As told by Sir Frederick Treves

*I*n the Mile End Road,* opposite to the London Hospital, there was (and possibly still is) a line of small shops. Among them was a vacant greengrocer's which was to let. The whole of the front of the shop, with the exception of the door, was hidden by a hanging sheet of canvas on which was the announcement that the Elephant Man was to be seen within and that the price of admission was twopence.

Painted on the canvas in primitive colors was a life-size portrait of the Elephant Man. This very crude production depicted a frightful creature that could only have been possible in a nightmare. It was the figure of a man with the characteristics of an elephant. The transfiguration was not far advanced. There was still more of the man than of the beast. This fact – that it was still human – was the most repellent attribute of the creature. There was nothing about it of the pitiableness of the misshapened or the deformed, nothing of the grotesqueness of the freak, but merely the loathing insinuation of a man being

---

*This was an error, a lapse of memory on the part of Treves. Whitechapel Road was and is the name of the road.

17

changed into an animal. Some palm trees in the background of the picture suggested a jungle and might have led the imaginative to assume that it was in this wild that the perverted object had roamed.

When I first became aware of this phenomenon the exhibition was closed, but a well-informed boy sought the proprietor in a public house, and I was granted a private view on payment of a shilling. The shop was empty and grey with dust. Some old tins and a few shrivelled potatoes occupied a shelf and some vague vegetable refuse the window. The light in the place was dim, being obscured by the painted placard outside. The far end of the shop – where I expect the late proprietor sat at a desk – was cut off by a curtain or rather by a red tablecloth suspended from a cord by a few rings. The room was cold and dank, for it was the month of November. The year, I might say, was 1884.

The showman pulled back the curtain and revealed a bent figure crouching on a stool and covered by a brown blanket. In front of it, on a tripod, was a large brick heated by a Bunsen burner. Over this the creature was huddled to warm itself. It never moved when the curtain was drawn back. Locked up in an empty shop and lit by the faint blue light of the gas jet, this hunched-up figure was the embodiment of loneliness. It might have been a captive in a cavern or a wizard watching for unholy manifestations in the ghostly flame. Outside the sun was shining and one could hear the footsteps of the passersby, a tune whistled by a boy and the companionable hum of traffic in the road.

The showman – speaking as if to a dog – called out harshly: "Stand up!" The thing arose slowly and let the blanket that covered its head and back fall to the ground.

There stood revealed the most disgusting specimen of humanity that I have ever seen. In the course of my profession I had come upon lamentable deformities of the face due to injury or disease, as well as mutilations and contortions of the body depending upon like causes; but at no time had I met with such a degraded or perverted version of a human being as this lone figure displayed.

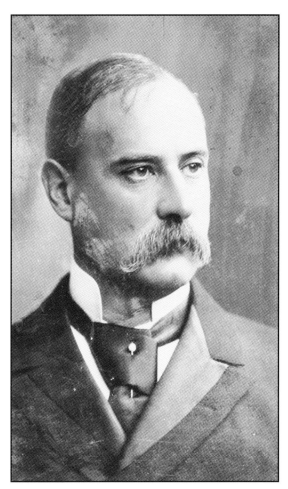

Figure 2. Sir Frederick Treves, the London surgeon who rescued the Elephant Man, as he appeared around the turn of the century. (Courtesy of the Library of The College of Physicians of Philadelphia)

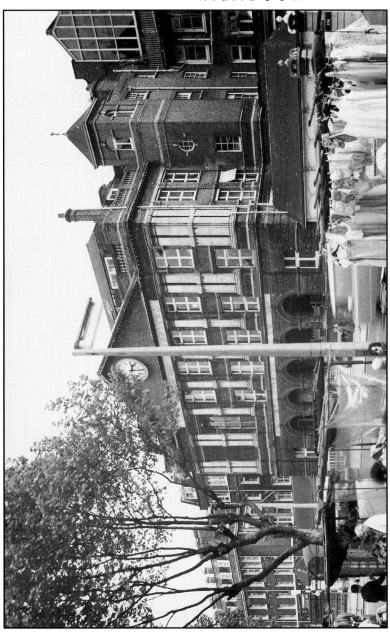

Figure 3.
Main front of
the London
Hospital from
the south side
of White-
chapel Road,
in 1970.

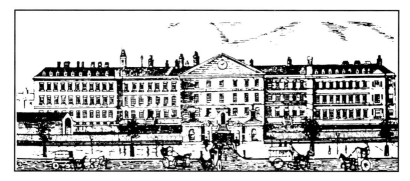

Figure 4. The London Hospital, as it appeared in the 1880s. (Courtesy of the London Hospital Medical College)

Figure 5. The London Hospital Medical College, as it looked in 1887. (Drawings from the *Illustrated London News*)

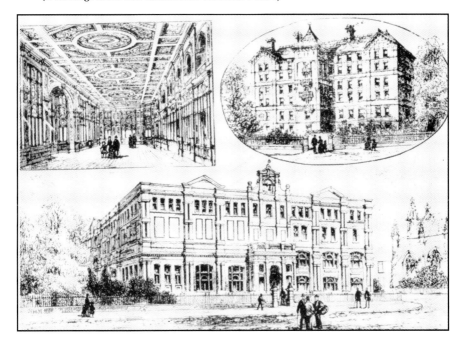

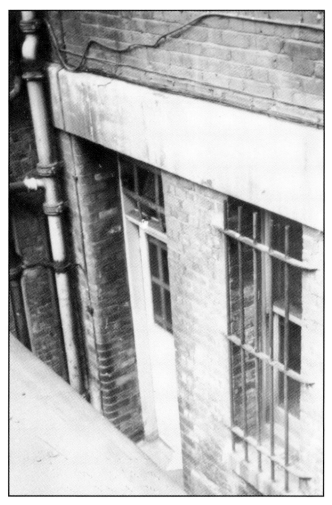

Figure 6. Entrance to Merrick's apartment – his "home," as he called it – in the London Hospital.

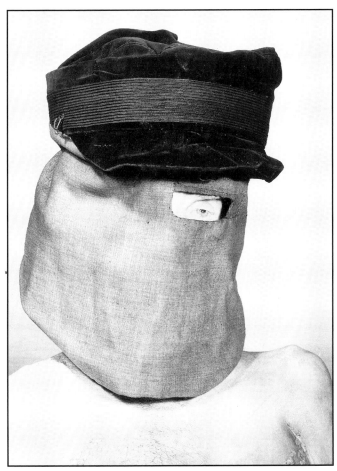

Figure 7. Joseph Merrick, the Elephant Man, with the cap and mask he wore on excursions outside his apartment in the London Hospital.

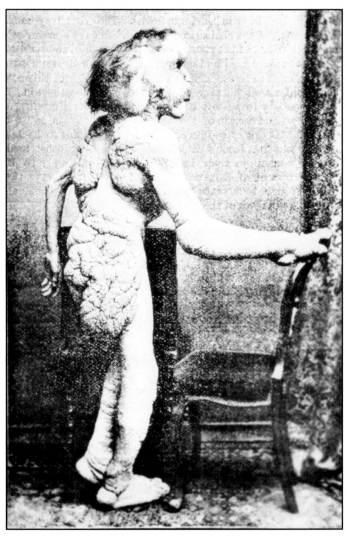

Figure 8. Merrick as he appeared some months before his death (From the British Medical Journal, Vol. 1, 1890, p. 916).

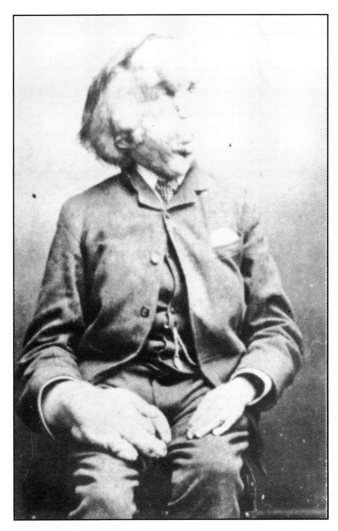

Figure 9. Merrick, dressed up, circa 1889, the year before his death.

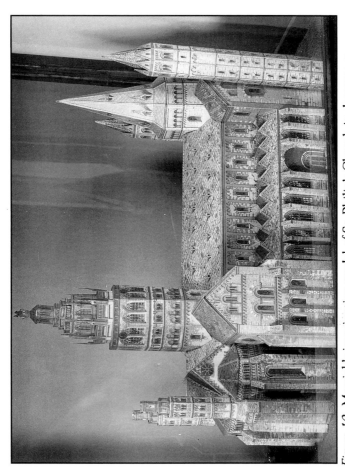

Figure 10. Merrick's imaginative model of St. Philip's Church in downtown London. Remarkably, he made the model, mostly with cardboard, using his one good hand. It is not clear where he acquired this skill, though he might have picked it up during one of his stints in the workhouse.

He was naked to the waist, his feet were bare, he wore a pair of threadbare trousers that had once belonged to some fat gentleman's dress suit.

From the intensified painting in the street I had imagined the Elephant Man to be of gigantic size. This, however, was a little man below the average height and made to look shorter by the bowing of his back.

The most striking feature about him was his enormous and misshapened head. From the brow there projected a huge bony mass like a loaf, while from the back of the head hung a bag of spongy, fungous-looking skin, the surface of which was comparable to brown cauliflower. On the top of the skull were a few long lank hairs. The osseous growth on the forehead almost occluded one eye. The circumference of the head was no less than that of the man's waist. From the upper jaw there projected another mass of bone. It protruded from the mouth like a pink stump, turning the upper lip inside out and making of the mouth a mere slobbering aperture. This growth from the jaw had been so exaggerated in the painting as to appear to be a rudimentary trunk or tusk. The nose was merely a lump of flesh, only recognizable as a nose from its position. The face was no more capable of expression than a block of gnarled wood. The back was horrible, because from it hung, as far down as the middle of the thigh, huge, sack-like masses of flesh covered by the same loathsome cauliflower skin.

The right arm was of enormous size and shapeless. It suggested the limb of the subject of elephantiasis. It was overgrown also with pendent masses of the same cauliflower-like skin.

The hand was large and clumsy – a fin or paddle rather than a hand. There was no distinction between the palm and the back. The thumb had the appearance of a radish, while the fingers might have been thick, tuberous roots. As a limb it was almost useless.

The other arm was remarkable by contrast. It was not only normal but was, moreover, a delicately shaped limb covered with fine skin and provided with a beautiful hand which any woman might have envied.

From the chest hung a bag of the same repulsive flesh. It was like a dewlap suspended from the neck of a lizard.

The lower limbs had the characters of the deformed arm. They were unwieldy, dropsical-looking and grossly misshapen.

To add a further burden to his trouble the wretched man, when a boy, developed hip disease, which had left him permanently lame, so that he could only walk with a stick. He was thus denied all means of escape from his tormentors. As he told me later, he could never run away.

One other feature must be mentioned to emphasize his isolation from his kind. Although he was already repellent enough, there arose from the fungous skin-growth with which he was almost covered a very sickening stench which was hard to tolerate.

From the showman I learnt nothing about the Elephant Man, except that he was English, that his name was John Merrick and that he was 21 years of age.

As at the time of my discovery of the Elephant Man I was the lecturer on anatomy at the Medical College opposite, I was anxious to examine him in detail and to prepare an account of his abnormalities. I therefore arranged with the showman that I should interview his strange exhibit in my room at the college.

I became at once conscious of a difficulty. The Elephant Man could not show himself in the streets. He would have been mobbed by the crowd and seized by the police. He was, in fact, as secluded from the world as the Man with the Iron Mask.

He had, however, a disguise, although it was almost as startling as he was himself. It consisted of a long black cloak which reached to the ground. Whence the cloak had been obtained I cannot imagine. I had only seen such a garment on the stage wrapped about the figure of a Venetian bravo. The recluse was provided with a pair of bag-like slippers in which to hide his deformed feet.

On his head was a cap of a kind that never before was seen. It was black like the cloak, had a wide peak, and the general outline of a yachting cap. As the circumference of Merrick's head was that of a man's waist, the size of this headgear may be imagined. From the attachment of the peak a grey flannel curtain hung in front of the face. In this mask was cut a wide horizontal slit through which the wearer could look out. This costume, worn by a bent man hobbling along with a stick, is probably the most remarkable and the most uncanny that has as yet been designed.

I arranged that Merrick should cross the road in a cab, and to insure his immediate admission to the college I gave him my card. This card was destined to play a critical part in Merrick's life.

I made a careful examination of my visitor, the result of which I embodied in a paper. I made little of the man himself. He was shy, confused, not a little frightened and evidently much cowed. Moreover, his speech was almost unintelligible. The great bony mass that projected from his mouth blurred his utterance and made the articulation of certain words impossible.

He returned in a cab to the place of exhibition, and I assumed that I had seen the last of him, especially as I found next day that the show had been forbidden by the police and that the shop was empty.

I supposed that Merrick was imbecile and had been imbecile from birth. The fact that his face was incapable of expression, that his speech was a mere spluttering and his attitude that of one whose mind was void of all emotions and concerns, gave grounds for this belief. The conviction was no doubt encouraged by the hope that his intellect was the blank I imagined it to be. That he could appreciate his position was unthinkable.

Here was a man in the heyday of youth who was so vilely deformed that everyone he met confronted him with a look of horror and disgust. He was taken about the country to be exhibited as a monstrosity and an object of loathing. He was shunned like a leper, housed like a wild beast, and got his only view of the world from a peephole in a showman's cart. He was, moreover, lame, had but one available arm, and could hardly make his utterances understood.

It was not until I came to know that Merrick was highly

intelligent, that he possessed an acute sensibility and – worse than all – a romantic imagination that I realized the overwhelming tragedy of his life.

The episode of the Elephant Man was, I imagined, closed; but I was fated to meet him again, two years later, under more dramatic conditions.

In England the showman and Merrick had been moved on from place to place by the police, who considered the exhibition degrading and among the things that could not be allowed. It was hoped that in the uncritical retreats of Mile End a more abiding peace would be found. But it was not to be. The official mind there, as elsewhere, very properly decreed that the public exposure of Merrick and his deformities transgressed the limits of decency. The show must close.

The showman, in despair, fled with his charge to the Continent. Whither he roamed at first I do not know, but he came finally to Brussels. His reception was discouraging. Brussels was firm; the exhibition was banned; it was brutal, indecent and immoral, and could not be permitted within the confines of Belgium.

Merrick was thus no longer of value. He was no longer a source of profitable entertainment. He was a burden. He must be gotten rid of. The elimination of Merrick was a simple matter. He could offer no resistance. He was as docile as a sick sheep. The impresario, having robbed Merrick of his paltry savings, gave him a ticket to London, saw him into the train and no doubt in parting condemned him to perdition.

His destination was Liverpool Street. The journey may be imagined. Merrick was in his alarming outdoor garb. He would be harried by an eager mob as he hobbled along the quay. They would run ahead to get a look at him. They would lift the hem of his cloak to peep at his body. He would try to hide in the train or in some dark corner of the boat, but never could he be free from that ring of curious eyes or from those whispers of fright and aversion.

He had but a few shillings in his pocket and nothing either to eat or drink on the way. A panic-dazed dog with a label on his collar would have received some sympathy and possibly some kindness. Merrick received none.

What was he to do when he reached London? He had not a friend in the world. He knew no more of London than he knew of Peking. How could he find a lodging, or what lodging-house keeper would dream of taking him in? All he wanted was to hide.

What most he dreaded were the open street and the gaze of his fellow-men. If even he crept into a cellar the horrid eyes and the still more dreaded whispers would follow him to its depths. Was there ever such a homecoming!

At Liverpool Street he was rescued from the crowd by the police and taken into the third-class waiting room. Here he sank on the floor in the darkest corner. The police were at a loss what to do with him. They had dealt with strange and mouldy tramps, but never with such an object as this. He could not explain himself. His speech was so maimed that he might as well have spoken in Arabic. He had, however, something with him which he produced with a ray of hope. It was my card.

The card simplified matters. It made it evident that this curious creature had an acquaintance and that the individual must be sent for. A messenger was dispatched to the London Hospital, which is comparatively near at hand. Fortunately I was in the building and returned at once with the messenger to the station.

In the waiting room I had some difficulty in making a way through the crowd, but there, on the floor in the corner, was Merrick.

He looked a mere heap. It seemed as if he had been thrown there like a bundle. He was so huddled up and so helpless-looking that he might have had both his arms and his legs broken. He seemed pleased to see me, but he was nearly done. The journey and want of food had reduced him to the last stage of exhaustion.

The police kindly helped him into a cab, and I drove him at once to the hospital. He appeared to be content, for he fell asleep almost as soon as he was seated and slept to the journey's end. He never said a word, but seemed to be satisfied that all was well.

In the attics of the hospital was an isolation ward with a single bed. It was used for emergency purposes – for a case of delirium tremens, for a man who had become suddenly insane or for a patient with an undetermined fever. Here the Elephant Man was deposited on a bed, was made comfortable and was supplied with food.

I had been guilty of an irregularity in admitting such a case, for the hospital was neither a refuge nor a home for incurables. Chronic cases were not accepted, but only those requiring active treatment, and Merrick was not in need of such treatment. I applied to the sympathetic chairman of the committee, Mr. Carr Gomm, who not only was good enough to approve my action but who agreed with me that Merrick must not again be turned out into the world.

Mr. Carr Gomm wrote a letter to *The Times* detailing the circumstances of the refugee and asking for money for his support. So generous is the English public that in a few days (I think in a week) enough money was forthcoming to maintain Merrick for life without any charge upon the hospital funds.

There chanced to be two empty rooms at the back of the hospital which were little used. They were on the ground floor, were out of the way, and opened upon a large courtyard called Bedstead Square, because here the iron beds were marshalled for cleaning and painting. The front room was converted into a bedsitting room and the smaller chamber into a bathroom.

The condition of Merrick's skin rendered a bath at least once a day a necessity, and I might here mention that with the use of a bath the unpleasant odor to which I have referred ceased to be noticeable.

Merrick took up his abode in the hospital in December of 1886. He had now something he had never dreamed of, never supposed to be possible: a home of his own for life.

I at once began to make myself acquainted with him and to endeavor to understand his mentality. It was a study of much interest. I very soon learned his speech so that I could talk freely with him. This afforded him great satisfaction, for, curiously enough, he had a passion for conversation, yet all his life had had no one to talk to. I, having then much leisure, saw him almost every day, and made a point of spending some two hours with him every Sunday morning, when he would chatter almost without ceasing.

It was unreasonable to expect one nurse to attend to him continuously, but there was no lack of temporary volunteers. As they did not all acquire his speech it came about that I had occasionally to act as an interpreter.

I found Merrick, as I have said, remarkably intelligent. He had learned to read and had become a most voracious reader. I think he had been taught when he was in the hospital with his diseased hip. His range of books was limited. The Bible and Prayer Book he knew intimately, but he had subsisted for the most part upon newspapers, or rather upon such fragments of old journals as he had chanced to pick up.

He had read a few stories and some elementary lesson books, but the delight of his life was a romance, especially a love romance. These tales were very real to him, as real as any narrative in the Bible, so that he would tell them to me as incidents in the lives of people who had lived.

In his outlook upon the world he was a child, yet a child with some of the tempestuous feelings of a man. He was an elemental being, so primitive that he might have spent the 23 years of his life immured in a cave.

Of his early days I could learn but little. He was very loathe to talk about the past. It was a nightmare, the shudder of which was still upon him. He was born, he believed, in or about Leicester. Of his father he knew absolutely nothing. Of his mother he had some memory. It was very faint and had, I think, been elaborated in his mind into something definite. Mothers figured in the tales he had read, and he wanted his mother to be one of those comfortable, lullaby-singing persons who are so lovable. In his subconscious mind there was apparently a germ of recollection in which someone figured who had been kind to him.

He clung to this conception and made it more real by invention, for since the day when he could toddle no one had been kind to him. As an infant he must have been repellent, although his deformities did not become gross until he had attained his full stature.

It was a favourite belief of his that his mother was beautiful. The fiction was, I am aware, one of his own making, but it was a great joy to him. His mother, lovely as she may have been, basely deserted him when he was very small, so small that his earliest clear memories were of the workhouse to which he had been taken. Worthless and inhuman as this mother was, he spoke of her with pride and even with reverence. Once, when referring to his own appearance, he said, "It *is* very strange, for, you see, mother was so beautiful."

The rest of Merrick's life up to the time that I met him at Liverpool Street Station was one dull record of degradation and squalor. He was dragged from town to town and from fair to fair as if he were a strange beast in a cage. A dozen times a day he would have to expose his nakedness and his piteous deformities before a gaping crowd who greeted him with such mutterings as, "Oh! What a horror! What a beast!"

He had had no childhood. He had had no boyhood. He had never experienced pleasure. He knew nothing of the joy of living nor of the fun of things. His sole idea of happiness was to creep into the dark and hide. Shut up alone in a booth, awaiting the next exhibition, how mocking must have sounded the laughter and merriment of the boys and girls outside who were enjoying the "fun of the fair"!

He had no past to look back upon and no future to look forward to. At the age of 20 he was a creature without hope. There was nothing in front of him but a vista of caravans creeping along a road, of rows of glaring show tents and of circles of staring eyes with, at the end, the spectacle of a broken man in a poor law infirmary.

Those who are interested in the evolution of character might speculate as to the effect of this brutish life upon a sensitive and intelligent man. It would be reasonable to surmise that he would become a spiteful and malignant misanthrope, swollen with venom and filled with hatred of his fellow-men, or, on the other hand, that he would degenerate into a despairing melancholic on the verge of idiocy. Merrick, however, was no such being. He had passed through the fire and had come out unscathed. His troubles had ennobled him. He showed himself to be a gentle, affectionate and lovable creature, as amiable as a happy woman, free from any trace of cynicism or resentment, without a grievance and without an unkind word for anyone. I have never heard him complain. I have never heard him deplore his ruined life or resent the treatment he had received at the hands of callous keepers.

His journey through life had been indeed along a *via dolorosa*, the road had been uphill all the way, and now, when the night was at its blackest and the way most steep, he had suddenly found himself, as it were, in a friendly inn, bright with light and warm with welcome. His gratitude to those about him was pathetic in its sincerity and eloquent in the childlike simplicity with which it was expressed.

As I learned more of this primitive creature I found that there were two anxieties which were prominent in his mind and which he revealed to me with diffidence. He was in the occupation of the rooms assigned to him and had been assured that he would be cared for to the end of his days. This, however, he found hard to realize, for he often asked me timidly to what place he would next be moved.

To understand his attitude it is necessary to remember that he had been moving on and moving on all his life. He knew no other state of existence. To him it was normal. He had passed from the workhouse to the hospital, from the hospital back to the workhouse, then from this town to that town or from one showman's caravan to another. He had never known a home nor any semblance of one. He had no possessions. His sole belongings, besides his clothes and some books, were the monstrous cap and the cloak. He was a wanderer, a pariah and an outcast. That his quarters at the hospital were his for life he could not understand. He could not rid his mind of the anxiety which had pursued him for so many years: *Where am I to be taken next?*

Another trouble was his dread of his fellow-men, his fear of people's eyes, the dread of being always stared at, the lash of the cruel mutterings of the crowd. In his home in Bedstead Square he was secluded; but now and then a thoughtless porter or a wardmaid would open his door to let curious friends have a peep at the Elephant Man. It therefore seemed to him as if the gaze of the world followed him still.

Influenced by these two obsessions he became, during his first few weeks at the hospital, curiously uneasy. At last, with much hesitation, he said to me one day:

"When I am next moved can I go to a blind asylum or to a lighthouse?"

He had read about blind asylums in the newspapers and was attracted by the thought of being among people who could not see. The lighthouse had another charm. It meant seclusion from the curious. There at least no one could open a door and peep in at him. There he would forget that he had once been the Elephant Man. There he would escape the vampire showman. He had never seen a lighthouse, but he had come upon a picture of the Eddystone, and it appeared to him that this lonely column of stone in the waste of the sea was such a home as he had longed for.

I had no great difficulty in ridding Merrick's mind of these ideas. I wanted him to get accustomed to his fellowmen, to become a human being himself and to be admitted to the communion of his kind. He appeared day by day less frightened, less haunted looking, less anxious to hide, less alarmed when he saw his door being opened. He got to know most of the people about the place, to be accustomed to their comings and goings, and to realize that they took no more than a friendly notice of him.

He could only go out after dark, and on fine nights ventured to take a walk in Bedstead Square clad in his black cloak and his cap. His greatest adventure was on one moonless evening when he walked alone as far as the hospital garden and back again.

To secure Merrick's recovery and to bring him, as it were, to life once more, it was necessary that he should make the acquaintance of men and women who would treat him as a normal and intelligent young man and not as a monster of deformity.

Women I felt to be more important than men in bringing about his transformation. Women were the more frightened of him, the more disgusted at his appearance and the more apt to give way to irrepressible expressions of aversion when they came into his presence. Moreover, Merrick had an admiration for women of such a kind that it attained almost to adoration. This was not the result of his personal experience. They were not real women but the products of his imagination. Among them was the beautiful mother surrounded, at a respectful distance, by heroines from the many romances he had read.

His first entry to the hospital was attended by a regrettable incident. He had been placed on the bed in the little attic, and a nurse had been instructed to bring him some food. Unfortunately, she had not been fully informed of Merrick's unusual appearance. As she entered the room she saw on the bed, propped up by white pillows, a monstrous figure as hideous as an Indian idol. She at once dropped the tray she was carrying and fled, with a shriek, through the door. Merrick was too weak to notice much, but the experience, I am afraid, was not new to him.

He was looked after by volunteer nurses whose ministrations were somewhat formal and constrained. Merrick, no doubt, was conscious that their service was purely official, that they were merely doing what they were told to do and that they were acting rather as automata than as women. They did not help him to feel that he was of their kind. On the contrary, they, without knowing it, made him aware that the gulf of separation was immeasurable.

Feeling this, I asked a friend of mine, a young and pretty widow, if she thought she could enter Merrick's room with a smile, wish him good morning and shake him by the hand. She said she could, and she did.

The effect upon poor Merrick was not quite what I had

expected. As he let go her hand he bent his head on his knees and sobbed until I thought he would never cease. The interview was over. He told me afterwards that this was the first woman who had ever smiled at him, and the first woman, in the whole of his life, who had shaken hands with him.

From this day the transformation of Merrick commenced and he began to change, little by little, from a hunted thing into a man. It was a wonderful change to witness and one that never ceased to fascinate me.

Merrick's case attracted much attention in the papers, with the result that he had a constant succession of visitors. Everybody wanted to see him. He must have been visited by almost every lady of note in the social world. They were all good enough to welcome him with a smile and to shake hands with him.

The Merrick whom I had found shivering behind a rag of a curtain in an empty shop was now conversant with duchesses and countesses and other ladies of high degree. They brought him presents, made his room bright with ornaments and pictures, and, what pleased him more than all, supplied him with books. He soon had a large library and most of his day was spent in reading. He was not the least spoiled, not the least puffed up. He never asked for anything, never presumed upon the kindness meted out to him, and was always humbly and profoundly grateful.

Above all, he lost his shyness. He liked to see his door pushed open and people to look in. He became acquainted with most of the frequenters of Bedstead Square, would chat with them at his window and show them some of his choicest presents. He improved in his speech, although to the end his utterances were not easy for strangers to understand. He was beginning, moreover, to be less conscious of his unsightliness, a little disposed to think it was, after all, not so very extreme. Possibly this was aided by the circumstance that I would not allow a mirror of any kind in his room.

The height of his social development was reached on an eventful day when Queen Alexandra – then Princess of Wales –

came to the hospital to pay him a special visit. With that kindness which marked every act of her life, the Queen entered Merrick's room smiling and shook him warmly by the hand. Merrick was transported with delight. This was beyond even his most extravagant dream. The Queen made many people happy, but I think no gracious act of hers ever caused such happiness as she brought into Merrick's room when she sat by his chair and talked to him as to a person she was glad to see.

Merrick, I may say, was now one of the most contented creatures I have chanced to meet. More than once he said to me:

"I am happy every hour of the day."

This was good to think upon when I recalled the half-dead heap of miserable humanity I had seen in the corner of the waiting room at Liverpool Street.

Most men of Merrick's age would have expressed their joy and sense of contentment by singing or whistling when they were alone. Unfortunately, poor Merrick's mouth was so deformed that he could neither whistle nor sing. He was satisfied to express himself by beating time upon the pillow to some tune that was ringing in his head. I have many times found him so occupied when I have entered his room unexpectedly.

One thing that always struck me as sad about Merrick was the fact that he could not smile. Whatever his delight might be, his face remained expressionless. He could weep, but he could not smile.

The Queen paid Merrick many visits and sent him every year a Christmas card with a message in her own handwriting. On one occasion she sent him a signed photograph of herself. Merrick, quite overcome, regarded it as a sacred object and would hardly allow me to touch it. He cried over it, and after it was framed had it put up in his room as a kind of icon.

I told him that he must write to Her Royal Highness to thank her for her goodness. This he was pleased to do, as he was very fond of writing letters, never before in his life having had anyone to write to. I allowed the letter to be dispatched unedited. It began "My dear Princess" and ended "Yours very sincerely."

Unorthodox as it was it was expressed in terms any courtier would have envied.

Other ladies followed the Queen's gracious example and sent their photographs to this delighted creature who had been all his life despised and rejected of men. His mantelpiece and table became so covered with photographs of handsome ladies, with dainty knick-knacks and pretty trifles that they may almost have befitted the apartment of an Adonis-like actor or of a famous tenor.

Through all these bewildering incidents and through the glamour of this great change Merrick still remained in many ways a mere child. He had all the invention of an imaginative boy or girl, the same love of "make-believe," the same instinct of "dressing up" and of personating heroic and impressive characters. This attitude of mind was illustrated by the following incident:

Benevolent visitors had given me, from time to time, sums of money to be expended for the comfort of the *ci-devant* Elephant Man. When one Christmas was approaching I asked Merrick what he would like me to purchase as a Christmas present. He rather startled me by saying shyly that he would like a dressing bag with silver fittings. He had seen a picture of such an article in an advertisement, which he had furtively preserved.

The association of a silver-fitted dressing bag with the poor wretch wrapped up in a dirty blanket in an empty shop was hard to comprehend. I fathomed the mystery in time, for Merrick made little secret of the fancies that haunted his boyish brain. Just as a small girl with a tinsel coronet and a window curtain for a train will realize the conception of a countess on her way to court, so Merrick loved to imagine himself a dandy and a young man about town. Mentally, no doubt, he had frequently "dressed up" for the part. He could "make-believe" with great effect, but he wanted something to render his fancied character more realistic. Hence the jaunty bag which was to assume the function of the toy coronet and the window curtain that could transform a mite with a pigtail into a countess.

As a theatrical "property" the dressing bag was ingenious,

since there was little else to give substance to the transformation. Merrick could not wear the silk hat of the dandy nor, indeed, any kind of hat. He could not adapt his body to the trimly cut coat. His deformity was such that he could wear neither collar nor tie, while in association with his bulbous feet the young blood's patent leather shoe was unthinkable. What was there left to make up the character? A lady had given him a ring to wear on his undeformed hand, and a noble lord had presented him with a very stylish walking stick. But these things, helpful as they were, were hardly sufficing.

The dressing bag, however, was distinctive, was explanatory and entirely characteristic. So the bag was obtained and Merrick the Elephant Man became, in the seclusion of his chamber, the Piccadilly exquisite, the young spark, the gallant, the "nut."

When I purchased the article I realized that as Merrick could never travel he could hardly want a dressing bag. He could not use the silver-backed brushes and the comb because he had no hair to brush. The ivory-handled razors were useless because he could not shave. The deformity of his mouth rendered an ordinary toothbrush of no avail, and as his monstrous lips could not hold a cigarette the cigarette case was a mockery. The silver shoehorn would be of no service in the putting on of his ungainly slippers, while the hat brush was quite unsuited to the peaked cap with its visor.

Still the bag was an emblem of the real swell and of the knockabout Don Juan of whom he had read. So every day Merrick laid out upon his table, with proud precision, the silver brushes, the razors, the shoehorn and the silver cigarette case, which I had taken care to fill with cigarettes. The contemplation of these gave him great pleasure, and such is the power of self-deception that they convinced him he was the "real thing."

I think there was just one shadow in Merrick's life. As I have already said, he had a lively imagination; he was romantic; he cherished an emotional regard for women, and his favorite pursuit was the reading of love stories. He fell in love – in a humble and devotional way – with, I think, every attractive lady he saw. He no doubt pictured himself the hero of many a passionate incident. His bodily deformity had left unmarred the instincts and feelings of his years. He was amorous. He would like to have been a lover, to have walked with the beloved object in the languorous shades of some beautiful garden and to have poured into her ear all the glowing utterances that he had rehearsed in his heart.

And yet – the pity of it! – imagine the feelings of such a youth when he saw nothing but a look of horror creep over the face of every girl whose eyes met his. I fancy when he talked of life among the blind there was a half-formed idea in his mind that he might be able to win the affection of a woman if only she were without eyes to see.

As Merrick developed he began to display certain modest ambitions in the direction of improving his mind and enlarging his knowledge of the world. He was as curious as a child and as eager to learn. There were so many things he wanted to know and to see. In the first place, he was anxious to view the interior of what he called "a real house," such a house as figured in many of the tales he knew, a house with a hall, a drawing room where guests were received and a diningroom with plates on the sideboard and with easy chairs into which the hero could "fling himself." The workhouse, the common lodginghouse and a variety of mean garrets were all the residences he knew.

To satisfy this wish I drove him up to my small house in Wimpole Street. He was absurdly interested, and examined everything in detail and with untiring curiosity. I could not show him the pampered menials and the powdered footmen of whom he had read, nor could I produce the white marble staircase of the mansion of romance nor the gilded mirrors and the brocaded divans which belong to that style of residence. I explained that the house was a modest dwelling of the Jane Austen type, and as he had read *Emma* he was content.

A more burning ambition of his was to go to the theatre. It was a project very difficult to satisfy. A popular pantomime was then in progress at Drury Lane Theatre. But the problem was how so conspicuous a being as the Elephant Man could be gotten there, and how he was to see the performance without attracting the notice of the audience and causing a panic or, at least, an unpleasant diversion.

The whole matter was most ingeniously carried through by that kindest of women and most able of actresses, Mrs. Kendal. She made the necessary arrangements with the lessee of the theatre. A box was obtained. Merrick was brought up in a carriage with drawn blinds and was allowed to make use of the royal entrance so as to reach the box by a private stair. I had begged three of the hospital sisters to don evening dress and to sit in the front row in order to "dress" the box, on the one hand, and to form a screen for Merrick on the other. Merrick and I occupied the back of the box, which was kept in shadow. All went well, and no one saw a figure, more monstrous than any on the stage, mount the staircase or cross the corridor.

One has often witnessed the unconstrained delight of a child at its first pantomime, but Merrick's rapture was much more intense as well as much more solemn. Here was a being with the brain of a man, the fancies of a youth and the imagination of a child. His attitude was not so much that of delight as of wonder and amazement. He was awed. He was enthralled. The spectacle left him speechless, so that if he were spoken to he took no heed. He often seemed to be panting for breath.

I could not help comparing him with a man of his own age in the stalls. This satiated individual was bored to distraction, would look wearily at the stage from time to time and then yawn as if he had not slept for nights; while at the same time Merrick was thrilled by a vision that was almost beyond his comprehension.

Merrick talked of this pantomime for weeks and weeks. To him, as to a child with the faculty of make-believe, everything was real; the palace was the home of kings, the princess was of royal blood, the fairies were as undoubted as the children in the street, while the dishes at the banquet were of unquestionable gold. He did not like to discuss it as a play but rather as a vision of some actual world. When this mood possessed him he would say:

"I wonder what the prince did after we left?" or "Do you think that poor man is still in the dungeon?"and so on and so on.

The splendor and display impressed him, but, I think, the ladies of the ballet took a still greater hold upon his fancy. He did not like the ogres and the giants, while the funny men impressed him as irreverent. Having no experience as a boy of romping and ragging, of practical jokes or of "larks," he had little sympathy with the doings of the clown, but, I think (moved by some mischievous instinct in his subconscious mind), he was pleased when the policeman was smacked in the face, knocked down and generally rendered undignified.

Later on another longing stirred the depths of Merrick's mind. It was a desire to see the country, a desire to live in some green secluded spot and there learn something about flowers and the ways of animals and birds. The country as viewed from a wagon on a dusty high road was all the country he knew. He had never wandered among the fields nor followed the windings of a wood. He had never climbed to the brow of a breezy down. He had never gathered flowers in a meadow. Since so much of his reading dealt with country life he was possessed by the wish to see the wonders of that life himself.

This involved a difficulty greater than that presented by a visit to the theatre. The project was, however, made possible on this occasion also by the kindness and generosity of a lady – Lady Knightley – who offered Merrick a holiday home in a cottage on her estate. Merrick was conveyed to the railway station in the usual way, but as he could hardly venture to appear on the platform the railway authorities were good enough to run a second-class carriage into a distant siding. To this point Merrick was driven and was placed in the carriage unobserved. The carriage, with the curtains drawn, was then attached to the mainline train.

He duly arrived at the cottage, but the housewife (like the nurse at the hospital) had not been made clearly aware of the unfortunate man's appearance. Thus it happened that when Merrick presented himself, his hostess, throwing her apron over her head, fled, gasping, to the fields. She affirmed that such a guest was beyond her powers of endurance, for when she saw him she was "that took" as to be in danger of being permanently "all of a tremble."

Merrick was then conveyed to a gamekeeper's cottage which was hidden from view and was close to the margin of a wood. The man and his wife were able to tolerate his presence. They treated him with the greatest kindness, and with them he spent the one supreme holiday of his life. He could roam where he pleased. He met no one on his wanderings, for the wood was preserved and denied to all but the gamekeeper and the forester.

There is no doubt that Merrick passed in this retreat the happiest time he had as yet experienced. He was alone in a land of wonders. The breath of the country passed over him like a healing wind. Into the silence of the wood the fearsome voice of the showman could never penetrate. No cruel eyes could peep at him through the friendly undergrowth. It seemed as if in this place of peace all stain had been wiped away from his sullied past. The Merrick who had once crouched terrified in the filthy shadows of a Mile End shop was now sitting in the sun, in a clearing among the trees, arranging a bunch of violets he had gathered.

His letters to me were the letters of a delighted and enthusiastic child. He gave an account of his trivial adventures, of the amazing things he had seen, and of the beautiful sounds he had heard. He had met with strange birds, had startled a hare from her form, had made friends with a fierce dog, and had watched the trout darting in a stream. He sent me some of the wild flowers he had picked. They were of the commonest and most familiar kind, but they were evidently regarded by him as rare and precious specimens.

He came back to London, to his quarters in Bedstead Square, much improved in health, pleased to be "home" again and to be once more among his books, his treasures and his many friends.

Some six months after Merrick's return from the country he was found dead in bed. This was in April of 1890. He was lying on his back as if asleep, and had evidently died suddenly and without a struggle, since not even the coverlet of the bed was disturbed. The method of his death was peculiar. So large and so heavy was his head that he could not sleep lying down. When he assumed the recumbent position the massive skull was inclined to drop backwards, with the result that he experienced no little distress.

The attitude he was compelled to assume when he slept was very strange. He sat up in bed with his back supported by pillows; his knees were drawn up, and his arms clasped round his legs, while his head rested on the points of his bent knees.

He often said to me that he wished he could lie down to sleep "like other people." I think on this last night he must, with some determination, have made the experiment. The pillow was soft, and the head, when placed on it, must have fallen backwards and caused a dislocation of the neck. Thus it came about that his death was due to the desire that had dominated his life: the pathetic but hopeless desire to be "like other people."

As a specimen of humanity, Merrick was ignoble and repulsive; but the spirit of Merrick, if it could be seen in the form of the living, would assume the figure of an upstanding and heroic man, smooth-browed and clean of limb, and with eyes that flashed undaunted courage.

His tortured journey had come to an end. All the way he, like another, had borne on his back a burden almost too grievous to bear. He had been plunged into the Slough of Despond, but with manly steps had gained the farther shore. He had been made "a spectacle to all men" in the heartless streets of Vanity Fair. He had been ill-treated and reviled and bespattered with the mud of Disdain. He had escaped the clutches of the Giant Despair, and at last had reached the "Place of Deliverance," where "his burden loosed from off his shoulders and fell from off his back, so that he saw it no more."

Chapter Five

Building On Treves' Story

*S*ir Frederick Treves' account of the Elephant Man is undoubtedly one of the most interesting and poignant on record. Since his essay was originally published, in 1923, additional information has been uncovered which further illuminates the tragic, intriguing life story of Joseph Merrick.

This newer information bears on minor and major points of the story, such as the fact that the Elephant Man is said to have been born a "perfect baby," free from any hint of deformity, that he had a brother and sister, that his mother loved and cared for him until he was nearly 11 years old, and that this gentle woman did not send him to the dreaded workhouse, as Treves had assumed.

Joseph Carey Merrick, who would later become known as "the Elephant Man," was born 5 August 1862 at 50 Lee Street, in the sub-district of East Leicester, in the County of Leicester. On his birth certificate his mother's name is entered as Mary Jane Merrick (née Potterton).

His father's name was Joseph Rockley Merrick. Mary Jane's

47

father was a farm laborer. Joseph Rockley's family had also been farm laborers.

Mary Jane is said to have been a cripple, but how this came about is not recorded. The story that she was somehow injured during the flight of a rogue elephant from a circus may or may not be true. It is known that for some time she was a teacher in a Baptist Sunday School.

Mary Jane Potterton and Joseph Rockley Merrick were married in the parish church of Thurmaston, several miles north of Leicester, on 29 December 1861. It has been suggested that Mary Jane may have been pregnant when she married. This, however, is a rather gratuitous judgment. The average duration of pregnancy is 266½ days. From the day of their marriage until Joseph Carey's birth 243 days had elapsed; in other words, a little less than three weeks of the average duration of pregnancy – well within the range of variation for normal healthy births.[5]

At the time of their marriage Mary Jane had been in service for some 13 years, and Joseph Rockley was employed as the driver of a brougham, a four-wheel cab. By the time his son, Joseph Carey, was born he had become a warehouseman and a factory engine-driver.

According to an article in the 27 December 1930 *Illustrated Leicester Chronicle*, by an anonymous writer who appears to have had an intimate acquaintance with the Merrick family, Joseph Carey was born a perfect baby. Merrick's mother first noticed that something was wrong when a swelling formed on her 21-month-old infant's lower lip. This grew progressively worse, and soon there were signs of involvement of other parts of the child's body. For the next nine years, until her death, Mary Jane devoted herself to the care of her suffering, deformed child.[6]

In his *Autobiography* Joseph Merrick says that his disorder "was not perceived much at birth, but began to develop itself when at the age of five years."

In 1866 Mary Jane gave birth to another son; he was named William Arthur. It was about this time that Joseph Carey fell and injured his left hip-joint; this soon became disordered and, added to his other miseries, left him lame for life, with one leg shorter than the other.

In September 1867 Mary Jane gave birth to a daughter, who was named Marion Elizabeth. A few days before Christmas 1870 little William Arthur died of scarlet fever. In the spring of 1873 Mary Jane developed broncho-pneumonia, and on 19 May, her thirty-sixth birthday, she died. Joseph Carey was then ten years and nine months old. It was a devastating blow to him. His mother's love and protectiveness was his all-embracing support, and that was now suddenly, catastrophically, at an end.

Left with two children to raise, with a job as a driver in a factory, and the owner of a small haberdashery shop to which Mary Jane had attended, Joseph Rockley decided to find accommodation for himself and his two children in the nearby home of a young widow, Mrs. Emma Wood Antill. Mrs. Antill had two young children of her own. On 3 December 1874 Joseph Rockley and Mrs. Antill were married – an event which proved a disaster for the 12-year-old Merrick.

Twelve was the customary age for children of the working classes to leave school. Mrs. Antill did not take kindly to her stepson; she found him a burden and soon made that clear to him. She demanded that young Joseph find immediate employment.

After much perseverance Merrick found work in a cigar factory. There he labored for nearly two years. By the end of that period the deformity of his right hand had progressed at such a rate that he was no longer able to roll the cigar leaves, and was discharged.

Whereupon his father obtained for him a hawker's license to peddle some of the smaller items from the haberdashery shop.

One can imagine the kind of reception Merrick received, knocking at door after door, offering his goods for sale. There were, possibly, some who were kind, and somehow he did manage to sell a few items. With the money he obtained he paid for meals which he took outside, for he could no longer endure the taunts and ill-treatment he received at "home." On one occasion upon his return to the house he received a severe beating from his father for having spent too much of his earnings on food.

That was the final betrayal. It seemed to him that his father had now gone over entirely to the enemy. He was 14 years of age and alone in a cruel world. There was nothing left for him to do but to leave the house and never return.

Completely on his own, young Merrick attempted to earn a living by hawking hosiery on the streets of Leicester. With such small sums as he earned he paid for an occasional meal and a bed at night in the poorest of the town's common lodging houses. Destitute, abandoned and abhorred, in pain and misery, each day was a night of fretful gloom through which no star of heaven would appear to light the way. He had become a vagrant. There were shelterless nights. All he could do would be to bide in helpless misery the silent morrow with no glimmer of hope to comfort him. But help was on the way.

Charles Merrick, Joseph's paternal uncle, learning of his plight, set out in search of him, and, finally having found him, persuaded him to come and live with him and his wife above his hairdressing shop. Here Joseph spent two fairly happy years, earning his keep by continuing to hawk mainly hosiery about the streets of Leicester.

During this period the tumors on his head and face continued to grow, adding to his already grotesque appearance. Wherever he went small crowds would gather and follow him, taunting him and otherwise creating a nuisance. This soon came to the attention of the licensing body, which, in the public interest, denied his application for renewal of his license.

Once more Merrick found himself deprived of a means of sustenance, this time in his uncle's household. His aunt was about to have a baby, and Merrick saw that this would put a burden and an extra strain on the family. In desperation he felt the only solution to the problem was the workhouse.

On the Monday after Christmas, 29 December 1879, at the age of 17, Merrick was admitted to the Leicester Union Workhouse. It was his last resort, the ultimate refuge of the hopeless and the abandoned. George Crabbe's description of the work-house of the Eighteenth Century still held true for that of the Nineteenth:[7]

> There children dwell who know no parents' care:
> Parents who know no Children's love, dwell there;
> Heart-broken Matrons on their joyless bed
> Forsaken Wives and Mothers never wed;
> Dejected Widows and unheeded tears,
> And crippled Age with more than childhood's fears;
> The Lame, the Blind, and, far the happiest they!
> The moping Idiot and the Madman gay.

It was Disraeli who said that no other term than that of imprisonment could be given to the confinement which the poor underwent in the union workhouse.

Treves was quite wrong in writing that Merrick had been sent to the workhouse by his mother. He should have known better than that, for no family in Victorian England would have sent anyone to the workhouse if it could possibly have been avoided. To the poor, more than any other class, the very word sounded like a knell, and justly conjured up visions of the bleakest of all dungeons – the last degradation to which the destitute and the hopeless were abandoned.

Merrick found the Leicester Union Workhouse no improve-ment upon the reputation that such institutions enjoyed. After three months of wretchedness there he signed himself out on 22 March 1880.

For two days Merrick vainly and dishearteningly attempted to find any sort of employment in what must have seemed to him a heartless world. The experiences he must have suffered during those two days, added to the realization that he would never be able to earn a living in the outside world, drove him back to the only shelter he knew would take him in, miserable and demean-ing though it was, the Leicester Union Workhouse. Here, once more, he found himself a victim of the archaic and inhuman Poor Laws of England. This time he remained in the workhouse for four years and eight months.

Toward the end of this period there had come to Leicester a popular comedian of the London and provincial music halls, Sam Torr. Sam had bought a hotel in town known as the Gladstone Vaults; to this he added a music hall. Merrick read of these events in the newspaper. He knew that music halls often showed all sorts of curiosities to pique the interest of the frequenters of such places, and in this he saw a possible way out of his misery. So, he wrote to Sam Torr offering himself for exhibition.

The amiable Torr called upon Merrick immediately. On meeting Merrick he had no doubt that he was a marketable attraction, but equally he had no doubt that no freak of any kind could attract a profitable audience for more than a week or so. Torr knew that such exhibits soon palled upon the public and therefore had to be changed frequently. He therefore asked Merrick whether he would mind travelling around the country under the auspices of himself and several of his friends in the same line of business. Merrick saw no objection to this, and so an agreement was signed, and Merrick signed himself out of the Leicester Union Workhouse on 29 August 1884, never to return.

Merrick lodged with Torr, and was now under the immediate charge of his employer and Mr. J. Ellis, one of the four members of the consortium of managers under whom Merrick was to work. Ellis was the proprietor of "The Living," a "Palace of Varieties at the Bee-Hive Vaults" in the neighboring town of Nottingham. It was at this time, in preparation for his exhibition under the management of Torr and Ellis, that Merrick wrote a brief autobiography of himself. (See Appendix 1.)

On the back cover of the eight-page *Autobiography* Ellis and Torr advertised their respective music halls, and we may assume they shared in the profits from the sale of the pamphlet with

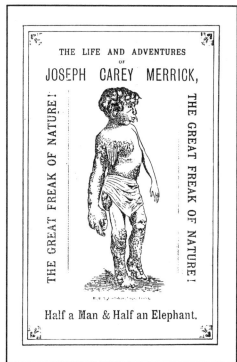

Fig. 11. The front and back covers of The *Autobiography* of Joseph Merrick, a piece written by Merrick to promote his exhibition in Europe in the 1880s.

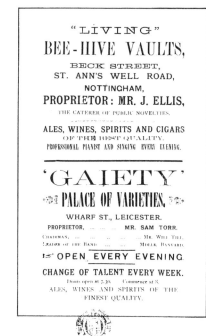

Merrick. There is every reason to believe that both Torr and Ellis treated Merrick with sympathy and understanding. Treves was quite wrong in assuming that all of Merrick's exhibitors were heartless exploiters.

One of Merrick's managers, Mr. Tom Norman, left an unpublished autobiography entitled "This is Tom Norman: Sixty-Five Years a Showman and Auctioneer," in which he writes, *apropos* of the two or more years that Merrick spent with him:

"I can honestly state that as far as his comfort was concerned whilst with us, no parent could have studied their child more than any or all the four of us studied Joseph Merrick . . . . The big majority of showmen are in the habit of treating their novelties as human beings, and in a large number of cases, as one of their own, and not like beasts."[8]

During his management under Tom Norman, Merrick managed to save some 50 pounds, a sizable sum in those days. When Treves encountered Merrick it was Tom Norman who was exhibiting him in the Whitechapel shop.

Already the days for such exhibitions were numbered; Victorian sentiment against such displays had risen to such a pitch that as soon as the newly formed governing body, the London County Council, went into action one of its first acts was to close down all freak shows and to declare them unlawful. This was in 1888, and since the Council's powers extended over all the parishes of London this meant the virtual end of freak shows over the whole of Greater London. Even before 1888 opposition to such shows had made itself strongly felt, by the conduct of the police in closing them and the support they received in doing so from the local magistrates.

Shortly after Treves exhibited Merrick before the Pathological Society of London the police closed the shop in which Norman was exhibiting Merrick. It was clear that the popularity of freak shows in England was coming to an end; this being so it was decided to send Merrick on a tour of the Continent.

This was carried out under the management of an impresario

said to be an Austrian. But on the Continent the show fared no better than in England as the police intervened at virtually every step. Show after show was closed down, and Merrick's Austrian showman, after stealing his 50 pounds, abandoned him in Brussels.

Destitute and alone in a land in which he could not understand a word of the language, and in which no one else could understand him, Merrick was somehow able to find a pawn shop and, with the money he obtained from the few things he had with him, he found his way to Ostend, where he was befriended by an Englishman named Wardell Cardew. With this gentleman's help he managed to get to Antwerp, and there he boarded the packet for Harwich, from which he could then take the train to Liverpool Street Station in London.

One can well imagine Merrick's sufferings during these seemingly endless days of torment, among which was the experience of being refused passage on one channel boat by a captain who feared that his presence on board might upset some of the passengers. It is a wonder that he could find a captain who would take him aboard, probably on the promise to make himself as invisible as possible. And so early in June 1886 at about seven in the morning Merrick arrived at Liverpool Street Station, only for a crowd soon to gather round him to gape and whisper among themselves at this strange apparition. He was clad in his black velvet cap, from which descended a linen flap that covered his face, with a single gap in it through which peered an eye, while from his shoulders descended a long black cloak down to his feet, which were encased in large rounded boot-like structures, the like of which they had never before encountered. The crowd and the center of its attention soon brought the police to the scene. The constables at once ushered Merrick into the third-class waiting room, to the darkest recess of which Merrick retired, to lie there in a hopeless, shapeless heap.

In response to questioning by the police, Merrick searching in the depths of his clothes produced a card with the name of

Frederick Treves and his address at the London Hospital. Since the hospital was not far distant from the railroad station and quite familiar to the police, one of them set off in search of Treves for such help as he might be able to give them. Fortunately, Treves was at the hospital, and from the description the policeman provided he at once recognized who the cause of the disturbance might be. So, hailing a cab, they together set off for Liverpool Street Station.

To say only that Merrick must have been glad to see Treves would be an understatement. Treves escorted the bewildered, though joyful Merrick out of the train station and accompanied him to the hospital, which was to become his home for the next three years or more.

Chapter Six

Life In
The London Hospital

hile Joseph Merrick was happy and relieved to have found shelter and compassion at the London Hospital, he was, nevertheless, unsettled in his new environment and apprehensive about his future. He found it difficult to believe that he had at long last come into safe harbor.

He feared that he might be moved on again, following the pattern of so much of his life when he was moved from place to place, town to town. He was anxious, timid, frightened, haunted-looking and alarmed when his door was opened.

These are the perfectly understandable reactions which any human being would develop after being subjected to years of maltreatment and debasement. Until he reached the safe haven of the London Hospital, he said that he had never before known what quiet and rest were.

As soon as Merrick became convinced that he had, indeed, come safely to rest, that his future was secure, that he no longer had anything to fear, and what is more, that he was a human being whom others valued and treated with respect, he lost all his defensive reactions. He became a changed man.

That he could say to Treves, more than once, "I am happy every hour of the day," must have been a most rewarding experience for Treves. At the same time this testifies to the recovery of Merrick from the awful trial of his former life.

One does not, of course, ever recover completely from the wounds inflicted by such an ordeal, but one can recover sufficiently to function healthily even though some scar tissue remains. This is what Merrick so eminently achieved.

Some six months after Merrick was brought to his new "home," the chairman of the hospital, Mr. Carr Gomm, wrote a letter to the editor of *The Times* of London appealing to the public for help in finding the Elephant Man a permanent residence, as well as providing some financial aid. His letter was published on 4 December 1886:

> To the Editor
> The Times
> London
>
> Sir,
>
> I am authorized to ask your powerful assistance in bringing to the notice of the public the following most exceptional case. There is now in a little room off one of our attic wards a man named Joseph Merrick, aged about 27, a native of Leicester, so dreadful a sight that he is unable even to come out by daylight to the garden.
>
> He has been called "the Elephant Man" on account of his terrible deformity. I will not shock your readers with any detailed description of his infirmities, but only one arm is available for work.
>
> Some 18 months ago, Mr. Treves, one of the surgeons of the London Hospital, saw him as he was exhibited in a room off the Whitechapel Road. The poor fellow was then covered by an old curtain, endeavouring to warm himself over a brick which was heated by a lamp. As soon as a sufficient number of pennies had been collected by the manager at the door, poor Merrick threw off his cur-

tain and exhibited himself in all his deformity.

He and the manager went halves in the net proceeds of his exhibition, until at last the police stopped the exhibition of his deformities as against public decency.

Unable to earn his livelihood by exhibiting himself any longer in England, he was persuaded to go over to Belgium, where he was taken in hand by an Austrian, who acted as his manager. Merrick managed in this way to save a sum of nearly 50 pounds, but the police there too kept him moving on, so that his life was a miserable and hunted one. One day, however, when the Austrian saw that the exhibition was pretty well played out, he decamped with poor Merrick's hardly-saved capital of 50 pounds, and left him alone and absolutely destitute in a foreign country.

Fortunately, however, he had something to pawn, by which he raised sufficient money to pay his passage back to England, for he felt that the only friend he had in the world was Mr. Treves of the London Hospital. He therefore, though with much difficulty, made his way there, for at every station and landing-place the curious crowd so thronged and dogged his steps that it was not an easy matter for him to get about. When he reached the London Hospital he had only the clothes in which he stood.

He has been taken in by our hospital, though there is, unfortunately, no hope of his cure, and the question now arises what is to be done with him in the future.

He has the greatest horror of the workhouse, nor is it possible, indeed, to send him into any place where he could not insure privacy, since his appearance is such that all shrink from him.

The Royal Hospital for Incurables and the British Home for Incurables both decline to take him in, even if sufficient funds were forthcoming to pay for him.

The police rightly prevent his being personally exhibited again. He cannot go out into the streets, as he is everywhere so mobbed that existence is impossible. He cannot, in justice to others, be put in the general ward of a workhouse, and from such, even if possible, he shrinks with the greatest horror. He ought not to be detained in our hospital (where he is occupying a private ward, and being treated with the greatest kindness – he says he has never before known in his life what quiet and rest were), since his case is incurable and not suited, therefore, to our overcrowded general hospital. The incurable hospitals refuse to take him in even if we paid for him in full, and the difficult question therefore remains what is to be done for him.

Terrible though his appearance is, so terrible indeed that women and nervous persons fly in terror from the sight of him, and that he is debarred from seeking to earn his livelihood in any ordinary way, yet he is superior in intelligence, can read and write, is quiet, gentle, not to say even refined in his mind. He occupies his time in the hospital by making with his one available hand little cardboard models, which he sends to the matron, doctor, and those who have been kind to him.

Through all the miserable vicissitudes of his life he has carried about a painting of his mother to show that she was a decent and presentable person, and as a memorial of the only one who was kind to him in life until he came under the kind care of the nursing staff of the London Hospital and the surgeon who has befriended him.

It is a case of singular affliction brought about through no fault of himself; he can but hope for quiet and privacy during a life which Mr. Treves assures me is not likely to be long.

Can any of your readers suggest to me some fitting place where he can be received? And then I feel sure that, when that is found, charitable people will come forward and enable me to provide him with such accommodation. In the meantime, though it is not the proper place for such an incurable case, the little room under the roof of our hospital...supplies him with all he wants.

The Master of the Temple on Advent Sunday preached an eloquent sermon on the subject of our Master's answer to the question, "Who did sin, this man or his parents, that he was born blind?" showing how one of the Creator's objects in permitting men to be born to a life of hopeless and miserable disability was that the works of God should be manifested in evoking the sympathy and kindly aid of those on whom such a heavy cross is not laid.

Some 76,000 patients a year pass through the doors of our hospital, but I have never before been authorized to invite public attention to any particular case, so it may well be believed that this case is exceptional.

Any communication about this should be addressed to myself or to the secretary at the London Hospital.

I have the honour to be, sir, yours obediently,

F. C. Carr Gomm
Chairman, London Hospital
November 30, 1886

The letter evoked many responses, particularly in the way of monetary donations and expressions of sympathy for this tragic figure. The money received as a result of the letter made it financially possible for Merrick to remain in the London Hospital under the watchful eye of Treves.

One cannot, without being deeply moved, read Treves' account of the occasion when, having persuaded a pretty young widow to visit Merrick and shake hands with him, Merrick was so overcome by the experience that he broke down and sobbed until Treves thought he would never cease. Apart from Merrick's mother the young widow was the first of her sex who had ever smiled at him, the first woman, in the whole of his life, who had ever shaken hands with him.

It was from that day that the transformation in Merrick commenced, and he began to feel like a normal human being. It was the first human contact he experienced with a woman since his mother.

From that day on Merrick was never failed for ladies of note in the social world to visit him, including the Princess of Wales (later Queen Alexandra), Lady Dorothy Neville, and others. The Prince of Wales (later Edward VII) also visited, as did the famous actor William Kendal. It was Mrs. Kendal who, though unable to visit Merrick, made it possible for him to see his first play, seated in the shadows of a private box, screened from view by a row of nurses sitting in front dressed in evening clothes. In spite of the immense trouble involved, Mrs. Kendal enabled Merrick to see other plays. It was also the brilliant and ever-kind Mrs. Kendal who, at her own expense, obtained the services of a teacher to instruct Merrick in the art of basket-making, an art at which Merrick soon excelled. (Mrs. Kendal died in 1935 at the age of 87, graced with honors and fondly remembered by everyone.)

From time to time the Prince of Wales sent Merrick game, and many gifts came to him from other personages. For three years and four months, with an occasional visit to the theater, with six-week stays in the country during the summer, Merrick lived happily in his rooms, his "home" as he called it, in the London Hospital.

Rising in the afternoon, he took his walks every day regularly in Bedstead Square, within the grounds of the hospital, and occupied himself with reading, model-making, and basket-making.

His health was good. He was happy. It would seem that he would now enjoy many happy years in comfort and security. But it was not to be.

On the night of 10 April 1890 Merrick took his usual walk, after which he retired for the evening. The next day at 1:30 in the afternoon the wardmaid brought him his dinner, which he did not eat. He appeared to be perfectly well at that time. Two hours later he was found dead.

Apart from his deformities and the increasing weight of his head, which he experienced more and more difficulty in holding erectly, Merrick was in relatively good health, although he is believed to have suffered from some undiagnosed cardiac condition as well as bronchitis. There was no reason to believe that he did not have at least several more years before him, though it was expected that he would die suddenly.

The fact that he did not touch his dinner suggests that he may have died shortly after the wardmaid left his room. Mr. Ashe, the house surgeon, who was called to the deceased at 3:30 that Friday afternoon, said at the inquest he believed that death was due to asphyxia, that the weight of the head, while Merrick was taking a natural sleep, overcame him and so suffocated him by causing pressure on the windpipe. Merrick died trying to be what he had ached to be all his life: normal.

As Treves explained, Merrick's customary mode of sleeping, owing to the great weight of his head, was in a seated position with his arms clasped around his legs and his chin resting on his knees. His oft-expressed wish to Treves that he might lie down to sleep "like other people," may have, on this final occasion, as Treves suggests, impelled him to try the experiment, with consequences that were fatal.

What probably happened is that his neck was dislocated, that the first neck vertebra (the atlas), as a consequence of the heavy head falling backward, slipped over the small tooth-like vertical process (the odontoid process) of the second neck vertebra, which, together with a ligament, normally keeps the first neck vertebra in place, and either ruptured or fatally compressed the spinal cord. I think it unlikely that asphyxia, as stated at the coroner's inquest, was the cause of death. Not even the coverlet of the bed was disturbed. There were no signs of a struggle for air. With rupture or compression of the cord at that level of the neck death would have been instantaneous.

The hospital staff and others who had come to know Joseph Merrick were quite saddened at the news of his death. Mr. Carr Gomm, the hospital's chairman, was moved to write a second letter to the editor of *The Times*, this one expressing gratitude to the newspaper and the public for their help and briefly reviewing Merrick's three and a half years as a resident of the hospital:

> To the Editor
> The Times
> London
>
> Sir,
>   In November, 1886, you were kind enough to insert in *The Times* a letter from me drawing attention to the case of Joseph Merrick, known as "the Elephant Man."
>   It was one of singular and exceptional misfortune. His physical deformities were of so appalling a character that

he was debarred from earning his livelihood in any other way than by being exhibited to the gaze of the curious.

This having been rightly interfered with by the police of this country, he was taken abroad by an Austrian adventurer, and exhibited at different places on the Continent. But one day his exhibitor, after stealing all the savings poor Merrick had carefully hoarded, decamped, leaving him destitute, friendless, and powerless in a foreign country.

With great difficulty he succeeded somehow or other in getting to the door of the London Hospital, where, through the kindness of one of our surgeons, he was sheltered for a time.

The difficulty then arose as to his future. No incurable hospital would take him in, he had a horror of the work-house, and no place where privacy was unattainable was to be thought of.... The rules and necessities of our general hospital forbade the fund and space – which are set apart solely for cure and healing – being utilized for the maintenance of a chronic case like this, however abnormal.

In this dilemma, while deterred by common humanity from evicting him again into the open street, I wrote to you, and from that moment all difficulty vanished. The sympathy of many was aroused, and, although no other fitting refuge offered, a sufficient sum was placed at my disposal, apart from the funds of the hospital, to maintain him for what did not promise to be a prolonged life.

As an exceptional case the committee agreed to allow him to remain in the hospital upon the annual payment of a sum equivalent to the average cost of an occupied bed.

Here, therefore, poor Merrick was enabled to pass the three and a half remaining years of his life in privacy and comfort. The authorities of the hospital, the medical staff, the chaplain, the sisters, and nurses united to alleviate as far as possible the misery of his existence, and he learnt to speak of his rooms at the hospital as his home.

There he received kindly visits from many, among them the highest in the land. His life was not without various interests and diversions: He was a great reader and was well supplied with books; through the kindness of a lady, one of the brightest ornaments of the theatrical profession, he was taught basket-making; and on more than one occasion he was taken to the play, which he witnessed from the seclusion of a private box.

He benefited much from the religious instruction of our chaplain, and Dr. Walsham How, then Bishop of Bedford, privately confirmed him. He was able by waiting in the vestry to hear and take part in the chapel services. The present chaplain tells me that on this Easter day, only five days before his death, Merrick was twice thus attending the chapel services, and in the morning partook of the Holy Communion. In the last conversation he had with him Merrick had expressed his feeling of deep gratitude for all that had been done for him here, and his acknowledgement of the mercy of God...in bringing him to this place.

Each year he much enjoyed a six weeks' outing in a quiet country cottage, but was always glad on his return to find himself once more "at home." In spite of all this indulgence he was quiet and unassuming, very grateful for all that was done for him, and conformed himself readily to the restrictions which were necessary.

I have given these details, thinking that those who sent money to use for his support would like to know how their charity was applied. Last Friday afternoon, though apparently in his usual health, he quietly passed away in sleep.

I have left in my hands a small balance of the money which has been sent to me from time to time for his support, and this I now propose, after paying certain gratuities, to hand over to the general funds of the hospital. This course, I believe, will be consonant with the wishes of the contributors.

It was the courtesy of *The Times* in inserting my letter in 1886 that procured for this afflicted man a comfortable protection during the last years of a previously wretched existence, and I desire to take this opportunity of thankfully acknowledging it.

I am, Sir, your obedient servant,

F.C.Carr Gomm
House Committee Room
London Hospital, April 15, 1890

It would seem that the Fates had prearranged Merrick's life course and allotted him a brief span of years. Saddled with a deformed body and grotesque appearance, crippled, lame, tortured and tormented, the compassionate interest of a young surgeon and a public subscription enabled him to spend the last few years of his life in a rapture that was all the more intensely felt by contrast with the squalor and misery of his former existence.

Merrick bore with courage and dignity the dreadful deformities and other ills with which he was afflicted. The nightmare existence he had led during the greater part of his life he put behind him. He never complained or spoke unkindly of those who had maltreated him.

His suffering, like a cleansing fire, seems to have brought him nearer to that human condition in which all the nonessentials of life having fallen away, only the essential goodness of man remained.

The life-changing power of affirmation

One of the more illuminating developments in Merrick's life while in the London Hospital is the transformation that was brought about in him by the kindnesses and affirmations of those around him.

During his stay in the hospital, Merrick was continually affirmed as a human being, worthy of love and respect, by Treves, the nurses, the hospital administrators, and especially by his many distinguished visitors, distinguished not only for their stations in life but also for their kindness.

With this reaffirmation of his humanity, a seemingly new

personality blossomed before their very eyes. It was the personality of someone who was beginning to feel secure, wanted, loved, self-confident, even happy.

This well-documented transformation of Joseph Merrick's personality is indeed an eloquent testimony to the potential life-changing power of affirmation.

Following his rescue by Treves, the sympathetic environment in which Merrick found himself enlivened his spirit and acted like an infusion of new blood into his body. Treves understood what the best treatment for Merrick's body and soul would be, and he set about providing it through his many connections as a distinguished surgeon.

From the Prince and Princess of Wales, the Duke of Cambridge, members of the aristocracy, and personalities of the theatre, Treves provided Merrick with a succession of fascinating visitors who took a genuine interest in him. Princess Alexandra not only visited Merrick but became a regular correspondent.

This host of new friends and supporters, coupled with the ongoing care and friendship of Treves, provided that affirmation of Merrick's humanity which he had longed for for many lonely years.

Merrick's humanity could have been lost earlier in life, for all practical purposes, had it not been for his mother's legacy of love. It saw him through the years of sorrow when he was regarded as a thing to be abhorred, a freak to be gaped at and rejected as belonging to the community of humankind. The inner strength which his mother's love gave him enabled him to survive the combination of his worsening bodily afflictions and the inhumanity of an unfeeling world.

To be rescued from that world by the kindness and sympathy of his newfound friends made it easier for him to bear his physical pain, and to be restored to that safe harbor of love which shaped him.

Chapter Seven

Setting The Record Straight

*W*hen Sir Frederick Treves wrote the story of the Elephant Man in 1922, he was nearly 70 years old, in ill-health, and straining to remember events that had occurred more than 30 years earlier. Treves had little else to go on but what a reluctant Joseph Merrick had told him, for, according to Treves, the past had been a nightmare for his beleaguered friend and therefore too painful to talk about.

Treves did what he could to get the story straight and complete, but the result of his attempt to reconstruct Merrick's past was to a great extent erroneous. Some things he appears to have forgotten completely, such as the small painting of Merrick's mother – his most prized possession – which corroborated Merrick's claim that his mother was a warm and "beautiful" woman. Other facts he managed to lose track of and therefore to misstate, such as Merrick's first name – an error that could have been avoided simply by checking with one of several documents which were readily accessible.

He also concluded incorrectly that Merrick was not loved by

his mother, that he was abandoned by her at an early age, and that those who managed the Elephant Man's exhibition in the freak shows were simply cruel and insensitive profiteers.

One of the oddest things about Treves' account of Merrick is his renaming of him. Merrick's name was Joseph Carey Merrick, and Joseph Merrick is the name by which he was known to virtually everyone who knew him.

Treves must have seen letters written by Merrick signed with his real name, and he may well have seen a copy of Merrick's *Autobiography*, in which he clearly states his name as "Joseph." Merrick's name was correctly recorded when he was given refuge in the London Hospital, and it was accurately stated in the letters to the editor of *The Times* that were written by Mr. Carr Gomm, the hospital's chairman. Yet, when he came to write of him 30 years later, Treves persisted in calling him "John."

By way of explanation, in view of Merrick's indistinct speech, it may be that Treves originally misheard the "Joseph" or "Joe" as "John" and simply began using that name without giving it a second thought.

In all of his published writings relating to Merrick, Treves consistently referred to him as "John," except in the final work to come from his pen, *The Elephant Man and Other Reminiscences*. In the typed manuscript he correctly called him "Joseph," but at the last moment before sending the manuscript off to the publisher crossed out "Joseph" and wrote above it "John" – the name which he had grown accustomed to using. This was in November of 1922.

Why Treves persisted in this error remains a bit of a mystery. But it may be that at the last moment he could not bring himself to admit that he had been using the wrong name for so long. Or it could be that he decided to stay with the use of "John" simply for the sake of consistency.

In his report of Merrick's disorder made to the Pathological Society of London on 17 March 1885, Treves states that Merrick "earned a living by exhibiting himself as 'the Elephant Man.' "

But this statement should not be taken to mean that Merrick did so on his own. It is very doubtful whether Merrick could ever have managed to exhibit himself without the aid of a manager or "impresario." Mr. Carr Gomm in his 1886 letter to *The Times* states that he and his manager "went halves in the net proceeds of his exhibition." And this appears to have been the arrangement into which Merrick entered with a series of "managers."

Treves writes of Merrick's dread of his fellowmen, of his fear of being stared at, and his great desire for seclusion from the curious – even to the extent of wanting to be sent to a home for the blind, so that no one could see his deformed shape. "His sole idea of happiness," writes Treves, "was to creep into the dark and hide."

This hardly suggests a person, however hard-pressed, who would willingly have exposed himself to the humiliations heaped upon him by men, women and children who would gape at him with horror and revulsion, as if he were some frightful monster. Nor is it conceivable that a creature as sensitive as Merrick, had he once tried such exposure to the crowd, would willingly have continued to do so. And yet hunger, which at first may have driven him to enter into such an arrangement, may have forced him to continue in the only way of life that was possible for him.

We have seen how Merrick came to place himself in the hands of showmen in order to escape from the workhouse. He was, indeed, lucky to find managers who were willing to take him on. Had he not done so he would have been forced to remain in the workhouse forever. How else could he have supported himself? How could he, whose articulation was so poor that he could hardly make himself understood, have made the necessary arrangements?

It is not a simple matter to exhibit oneself. Where could he have gone? Who would have taken him in? The sight he presented, with his long black cloak and the hood over his head, would have been frightening enough to cause every door to be closed against this apparition. Because of his appearance, so the 1886 account in the *British Medical Journal* reports, a steamboat captain refused to take him as a passenger. Even the Royal Hospital for Incurables and the Home for Incurables in London declined to take him in when, in 1886, he was finally rescued by Treves.

Such frustrations and humiliations were his daily fare. In some ways, then, he was better off being in the charge of a custodian, rather than having to attempt to shift for himself. Merrick almost certainly was aware of this, for the only alternatives before him were in this way to remain in the keeping of a manager or be altogether abandoned to his own helpless self. There was always the workhouse, but to this Merrick would never have returned voluntarily.

There was no possible means by which Merrick could have supported himself in Victorian England. It was difficult enough for normal men of the working classes to manage even so much as to subsist, and large numbers of them failed to do so. Merrick voluntarily entered into the arrangement with Mr. Torr to act as his manager, to be exhibited as "the Elephant Man" in return for a share of the profits and his bed and board. Once embarked upon this course, repellent as it must have been to him, Merrick saw no other way out.

What saved Merrick for the few happy years he was finally to enjoy was the police banning of such indecent exhibitions of a pitiful human being. He then became no longer profitable, and so, writes Treves, "The impresario, having robbed Merrick of his paltry savings, gave him a ticket to London, saw him into the train and no doubt in parting condemned him to perdition."

On the face of it, this is difficult to accept. I find it hard to understand why the "impresario" who had been profiting from the exhibition of Merrick would not have abandoned him altogether, especially after stealing his money. Why go to the trouble and expense of paying for his ticket to London, and seeing him into the train? Can it be that he was not altogether lacking in human feeling? Or is it possible that he was forced by the police to pay for the deportation of Merrick and required to see him safely placed on the train?

There is, in any case, another account of these events. This was given by Mr. Carr Gomm in his 1886 letter to *The Times*. In this communication we learn, "(Merrick) was persuaded to go over to Belgium, where he was taken in hand by an Austrian, who acted as his manager . . . . But the police, there too, kept him moving on." The manager, seeing that the exhibition was pretty nearly played out, decamped with nearly 50 pounds of Merrick's life savings, "and left him alone and absolutely destitute in a foreign country." Knowing no language but his own, and hardly being able to make himself understood in it, Merrick nevertheless managed to pawn something, and in this manner was able to raise enough money to pay his passage back to London.

In fact, what seems to have occurred is that by a stroke of good luck Merrick came to the attention of an English doctor in Ostend. This was Wardell Cardew, who happened to be a friend of the Kendals, who would later befriend Merrick and make elaborate arrangements for him to go to the theatre from time to time.

In a letter to W. H. Kendal, referring to Merrick, Cardew wrote, "I have had the most awful case in my care at Ostend."

Apparently he literally rescued Merrick, gave him shelter, and arranged for his return to England. Cardew played a role in Merrick's permanent settlement at the London Hospital, and also in helping to fund his support there.

Treves writes of Merrick that in his outlook upon the world he was a child, "an elemental being, so primitive that he might have spent the 23 years of his life [up to the time he came to rest in the London Hospital] immured in a cave."

Merrick was undoubtedly limited in his horizons, and possibly "primitive" in the sense that he had not matured in many of the traits that a normally socialized man develops, but he was scarcely "an elemental being."

That he was in some ways a simple person is attested by the fact that in order to account for his condition he either accepted from others or created for himself the story of a fright his mother had received shortly before his birth from having been injured by an elephant at a circus.

It is by no means surprising that Merrick should have clung to this belief. He needed some explanation for his condition, if only for himself, and this was better than most. It is quite understandable that a deformity which defied the abilities of the best physicians to explain should, in Merrick's unsophisticated mind, have found so clear and convincing a resolution.[9]

But this simplicity did not distinguish the whole of Merrick's character. His self-discipline and his skill at constructing his cardboard models, to name only two traits, show a being capable of more than "simplicity."

Treves states, "Since the day when he could toddle no one had been kind to him." If this were true then Merrick would, indeed, constitute an outstanding example of the constitutional ability of some children to resist the damaging effects of a lack-love infancy. But by "toddle" Merrick probably meant from the day he could remember. This could scarcely have been earlier than six or more years.

It, therefore, still remains a strong possibility that up to that time and beyond he received an adequate amount of mothering. Indeed, the evidence, as I have suggested, seems to point very much in this direction: that Merrick as a child received much love from his mother, and that it is highly unlikely that from birth onward he experienced nothing but an unbroken history of deprivation.

This is what I wrote when I had nothing more to rely on than what Treves had said, and because all the evidence with which I was familiar concerning the development of a child's personality could not be reconciled with Treves' statements. This was, of course, well before the facts revealed by Howell and Ford had become available, in their book, *The True History Of The Elephant Man*. Indeed, Merrick's mother died, as we have noted, when he was two to three months short of his eleventh birthday.

Treves was fully aware of the dramatic story he had to tell, and I cannot help but feel that he may well have exaggerated somewhat when he said that Merrick had neither childhood nor boyhood, and that he never experienced pleasure.

Certainly Merrick could never have enjoyed the kind of childhood and boyhood that normal children experience. Certainly he must have suffered keenly from the awareness that he was not like others, that he was to others a repellent creature. It is quite clear to me that he must have received a great deal of love from his mother, and that he took some pleasure, at least, in reading and doing the things with his one good hand that he was capable of doing.

Had Merrick suffered a life of as total deprivation as Treves suggests, his story would, in fact, be utterly mystifying, for his personality would then be wholly inexplicable.

From all we know of the development of human character, Merrick's personality could not have been what it was had he suffered from a lack-love infancy and childhood. Either our theory and observation of human development are wrong or Merrick would constitute an extraordinary exception to the rule. On the contrary, his case appears to confirm the rule, for no one could possibly have borne the torment of his later years and emerged from them as Merrick did had he not been fortified by the early experience of something more than a perfunctory love.

Chapter Eight

The Vindication
Of Mary Jane Merrick

*O*f the several errors Treves made in his account of the Elephant Man, the most unfortunate was his conjecture concerning Joseph Merrick's mother and the important role she played in the outcome of his character and personality.

Though Merrick often spoke of his mother as "beautiful," Treves dismissed this as a fiction of his imagination, a comforting thought that was a great joy to him, but nothing more. In so doing, Treves overlooked, or forgot, Merrick's most prized possession, a small painting of his mother – an item Treves surely would have seen on more than one occasion.

In reconstructing Merrick's life Treves persuaded himself that Merrick really had no recollection of his mother or indeed of his father.

"In his subconscious mind," Treves wrote, "there was apparently a germ of recollection in which someone figured who had been kind to him. He clung to this conception and made it more real by invention, for since the day he could toddle no one had been kind to him."

Treves could not have been more wrong, for the fact is that Merrick's mother cared for him until he was nearly eleven years of age. The portrait was more than "a germ of recollection;" to Merrick it *was* his mother – a mother of whom Merrick spoke, as Treves notes, with pride and reverence.

That Treves so completely forgot about the portrait may well mean that he had already made up his mind about Merrick's mother, and that Merrick's attachment to the painting was incompatible with the theory he chose to embrace concerning her.

The Nineteenth Century was not kind in its judgment of women, so it was not difficult for Treves to fall into a censorious view of a woman who he erroneously assumed had placed her child in a workhouse.

From Merrick's feeling for his mother and his own amiable nature there can be little doubt that Mary Jane Merrick was a loving mother. For a time she served as a Baptist Sunday School teacher, who we may surmise almost certainly saw to it that her son read the Bible and the Prayer Book, both of which he knew intimately.

What gave Merrick the strength to sustain his awful plight was almost certainly the gift of his mother's love, a benison without which he would have foundered. The pain, the torment, and the daily humiliations he suffered, he weathered with courage and fortitude.

Treves wrote of the kindliness of Merrick's character, indeed, of his nobility, and his abstention from ever speaking of the cruelty and pain he had suffered.

"As a specimen of humanity, Merrick was ignoble and repulsive; but the spirit of Merrick, if it could be seen in the form of the living, would assume the figure of an upstanding and heroic man, smooth-browed and clean of limb, and with eyes that flashed undaunted courage."

Precisely.   What struck me when I read these words in

Treves' description of Merrick's character was its incompatibil-
ity with his theory that Mary Jane Merrick had abandoned her
child at an early age to the Leicester Workhouse. It seemed to
me that Merrick must have received a good deal of love, especially during those critical years following birth.

Although I was a student of psychology in the early '20s,
there was no scientific research, and even less proof, of the
fundamental importance of maternal love for the healthy mental
development of the infant. This was not to come until the '40s
and '50s. The really fundamental work which proved the case
for maternal care was John Bowlby's *Maternal Care and Mental Health,* published by the World Health Organization at
Geneva in 1951, and reinforced by my survey of the evidence in
1955.[10]

Bowlby's book surveyed the whole of the relevant research
proving the indispensable necessity of maternal care for the
healthy mental development of the child to grow and develop
into a mentally healthy adult.

A short definition of mental health is the ability to love, to
work, to play, and to think soundly.

By love is meant the ability to communicate to the other, by
demonstrative acts, one's profound involvement in their welfare, such that you give them all the support, succor, stimulation, and encouragement for their healthy growth and development;
that they can always depend upon you standing by; that you will
never commit the supreme treason of letting them down when
they are in need; that you will always be there to respond to their
need; that you will help them fulfill themselves by nurturing and
encouraging them to realize all the potentialities that are within
them for becoming good and loving human beings, who will live
as if to live and love were one, loving others *more* than one
loves oneself.

It should be clear that this description of love is precisely
what a loving mother does for her child from birth, even before,
and onwards.

The love a mother gives her child constitutes the pattern and the basic patent by which we are designed to grow and develop all the days of our lives. Love is characterized by a wisdom that not even wisdom can replace. It is this love that made Joseph Merrick – in spite of the dreadful physical deformities from which he suffered – the loving spirit that he became, for when one is loved one grows spiritually.

Love is the greatest gift that one human being can make to another, and this is undoubtedly the gift from his mother that made Joseph Merrick what he became.

The ability to work is another essential component of mental health. Work is purposeful activity, mental or physical effort designed to do or make something. In Merrick's development it is highly probable that he worked well and enjoyed it, judging from his skill in the creation of a model cathedral from pieces of cardboard and colored papers. This is really quite beautiful, and when one considers it was all done with one hand, quite remarkable in and of itself.

It suggests that the young Merrick was encouraged to work at creating things of various sorts, that he enjoyed work, and that this helped him achieve a creative, self-healing harmony.

The habit of work can become a pleasure to which one looks forward with eagerness. Founded early in life work makes easier everything else one does later in life. Even though work may often involve burdensome and troubling effort, it is also a discipline which one comes to experience as a genuine part of the pleasure one takes in satisfactorily completing a task.

We may readily see how such a combination of challenges would have contributed to Merrick's ability to respond to them, as well as to the disorder which affected him. The harmony of both love and work gave him the spiritual strength he needed to meet these challenges – and to conquer them.

Treves' failure to figure out the source of Merrick's spiritual strength may appear strange, but for this he cannot be reproached, for he grew up in a society in which undemonstrativeness was the rule, a buttoned-up society, drunk on propriety, in which sensitivity to human need was strongly discouraged and any show of untoward feeling was considered ill-bred.

As E. M. Forster observed in 1920 in his brilliant essay, "Notes on the English Character," (in *Abinger Harvest.* New York: Harcourt, Brace, 1936, p.5.):

"It is not that the Englishman can't feel – it is that he is afraid to feel. He has been taught at . . . school that feeling is bad form. He must not express great joy or sorrow . . . . He must bottle up his emotions, or let them out only on a very special occasion."

In 1845 Benjamin Disraeli, in his novel *Sibyl,* called it "the English way." In 1816 Jane Austen in her novel *Emma* had used exactly the same words to describe the suppression, under a mask of calmness, of any form of feeling. The uncomfortableness felt at any display of affection made for unhappy marriages, the slighting of children, and a general inability to relate to others in anything other than an uninvolved kind of "cold fish" civility.

Entangled in such a web of social constraints, in which human beings were literally put out of touch with one another, it was difficult to extricate oneself.

Even so, Treves was clearly fascinated by the mystery of the Elephant Man's personality, as is evident in his writings:

> Those who are interested in the evolution of character might speculate as to the effect of this brutish life upon a sensitive and intelligent man. It would be reasonable to surmise that he would become a spiteful and malignant misanthrope, swollen with venom and filled with hatred of his fellow-men, or, on the other hand, that he would degenerate into a despairing melancholic on the verge of idiocy. Merrick, however, was no such being. He had passed though the fire and had come out unscathed. His troubles had ennobled him. He showed himself to be a gentle, affectionate and lovable creature, as amiable as a happy woman, free from any trace of cynicism or resentment, without a grievance and without an unkind word for anyone.

Indeed, Treves was keenly aware of the mystery of Joseph Merrick's character and personality. And while he was unable to arrive at the correct answer, he was at least able to formulate the question:

How could a creature so maltreated by Fate, so shockingly deformed and constantly racked by pain, so brutally treated by his fellowmen, have managed, in spite of everything, to emerge so unscarred, indeed, with so gentle, kind and generous a personality?

The answer can almost certainly be found, more than anywhere else, in the person of Mary Jane Merrick, his mother, and in the loving manner in which she reared and nurtured him.

Chapter Nine

The Supreme Importance Of A Mother's Love

*T*here is an ancient Middle Eastern saying that since God could not be everywhere he created mothers. This is a most beautiful and profound statement of a truth that is in every respect universally true and meaningful. It almost certainly represents the recollection of an age-old belief honoring the mother, the Great Mother, celebrating her role in the creation of humanity.[11]

The role of the mother's love in the behavioral development of the child is a major one, to put it mildly. It is *the* critical role in the whole process of children growing up to be healthy, loving human beings.

This is what I dimly understood when I read Sir Frederick Treves' *The Elephant Man and Other Reminiscences* late in 1923, shortly after its publication. I was led to the book from a review I had read while going through the literature in the student lounge at college. The review intrigued me, so I borrowed a copy of the book from the bookstore nearby.

The first story in the book was of the Elephant Man. It was 12 pages long, and it was fascinating, a moving and dramatic account of this hideously deformed young man who had been an outcast among his fellowmen, rejected, loathed, and exhibited as a freak for the crowd to gape at and revile. And despite his deformities and maltreatment, this Elephant Man had turned out to be a gentle, unembittered, loving human being.

How could this possibly be?

Of the early days of Joseph Merrick, the Elephant Man, Treves confessed that he could learn little. He believed they must have been a nightmare. Writing some 30 years after encountering the Elephant Man, Treves attempted to reconstruct those early days in Merrick's life as follows:

> Of his father he knew absolutely nothing. Of his mother he had some memory. It was very faint and had, I think, been elaborated in his mind into something definite. Mothers figured in the tales he had read, and he wanted his mother to be one of those comfortable lullaby-singing persons who are so lovable. In his subconscious mind there was apparently a germ of recollection in which someone figured who had been kind to him. He clung to this conception and made it more real by invention, for since the day he could toddle no one had been kind to him. As an infant he must have been repellent, although his deformities did not become gross until he had attained his full stature.
>
> It was a favourite belief of his that his mother was beautiful. The fiction was, I am aware, one of his own making, but it was a great joy to him. His mother, lovely as she may have been, basely deserted him when he was very small, so small that his earliest clear memories were of the workhouse to which he had been taken. Worthless and inhuman as this mother was, he spoke of her with pride and even with reverence. Once, when referring to his own appearance, he said, "It *is* very strange, for, you see, mother was so beautiful."

The curious thing here is that the only property that Merrick possessed and carried with him wherever he went was a small portrait of his mother. Merrick had undoubtedly shown it to Treves, who 30 years later, when he wrote his essay on Merrick, had apparently forgotten it. What is significant here is the love that Merrick expressed when, with deep feeling, he described his mother as beautiful; for, as we shall see, she must, in every sense of the word, have lived up to his view of her.

Treves' two paragraphs on Merrick's early days seemed to me utterly incompatible with Merrick's lovable personality. It was quite clear to me that something was awry with what Treves tried to put together of Merrick's history. Treves was a kind and sympathetic man, and if it had not been for him there would have been no rescue of "the half dead heap of miserable humanity." Merrick's fate would almost certainly have been very different from the heartwarming years he spent in the guardianship of Treves. Treves grew fond of Merrick and admired him, and yet failed to understand how Merrick came to be the lovable character that he was.

When I came to write my book on the Elephant Man, first published in 1971, I had already for 40 years been thoroughly immersed in the literature of child growth and development, as well as teaching it at The New School for Social Research, New York University, Harvard, Rutgers, and Princeton. I was, therefore, well-equipped to deal with the problems presented by Treves' account of the Elephant Man.

Even so, I found that I had taken a great deal that he had written for granted. But by far the most important conclusion for me was that Treves was probably completely wrong in assuming that Merrick's mother had abandoned him at an early age.

Treves is not to be condemned for his assumption, for the necessary scientific evidence which would have led him to another conclusion was simply not available in his day. That evidence, in the form of the numerous studies on maternal-infant relationships, together with the facts as revealed in Howell and

Ford's admirable book, *The True History of the Elephant Man*, published in 1980, fully corroborated the conclusion I had ventured many years earlier, namely, that the loving Joseph Merrick must have had a loving mother – a woman who cared for and nurtured him throughout his childhood, and not one who would have abandoned him at the tender age of three.

This is one of the great lessons that the Elephant Man story has to teach concerning love, namely, the supreme importance of a mother's love for her child.

Women everywhere, from the beginning of time, have known what it means to carry a child under one's heart, and after nine months to give birth to it.

The basic plan of the mother-infant relationship, from conception to birth, and onward, is that the loving behavior of the mother and child for one another confers survival and growth benefits upon each other. In this beautiful mother-and-child interconnectedness and interaction the basic pattern is laid out for humanity to follow toward the achievement of healthy growth and development, that is, to live as if to live and to love were one and the same.

The whole of humanity's experience testifies to the fact that when the child is loved it will itself grow up to be a loving person. Conversely, when a baby is not loved, if it survives, it will fail to grow and develop as a loving individual – simply because it has not learned to love.

The most important of all the basic needs with which the baby is endowed is the need for love – not simply to be loved, but to love others as well. This potentiality or predisposition is one of great power, but it will not develop unless it is animated by the stimulation and sustenance of love by being loved.

By love is meant to confer survival benefits in a creatively enlarging manner upon the other. And no one is better able to do this than mother and child for each other.

It is unfortunate that until recently this was not understood, largely because the supreme arbiters in these matters were men, particularly physicians and other males in positions of authority. Women as a whole intuitively understood the nature of this supremely natural bond, and no one better than the old-fashioned midwife who in the Twentieth Century virtually vanished from the scene (and who is now, happily, making a comeback).

But, the medical profession managed to persuade the world that pregnancy and birth were best treated in a hospital. Unfortunately, though, in institutions for foundlings and abandoned children the mortality rates were found to be phenomenally high.

At a meeting of the American Pediatric Society held in Philadelphia in 1914 Dr. Henry D. Chapin, a leading pediatrician of his day, in a report on the care of infants in ten cities in the United States, stated he found that in all but one such institution every infant under two years of age died.[12]   From their own experience a number of discussants of Dr. Chapin's report fully corroborated his findings.   Dr. R. Hamil remarked with grim irony:

"I had the honor to be connected with an institution in...Philadelphia in which the mortality among infants under one year of age, when admitted to the institution and retained there for any length of time, was 100 percent."

Dr. R. T. Southworth added:

"I can give an instance from an institution in New York City in which, on account of the very considerable mortality among the infants admitted, it was customary to enter the condition of every infant on the admission card as hopeless. That covered all subsequent happenings."

And so the story went, in Europe as well as in America. It was as if infants in institutions were expected to die there. No one knew what they died of, so it had to be given a name. It was called *"marasmas,"* the Greek word for "wasting away." Later it was called "infant debility," and today it still lingers on as "failure to thrive."

One of the striking things about the newborn, during the first two weeks following birth, is its striving for the satisfaction of its most important need, its hunger, for love. It was the lack of satisfaction of this most pressing of all the humanizing needs, the need for love, that was responsible for the wasting away and early death of the institutionalized infants.

The only way we learn to love is by being loved. It is a basic need, like the need for communication, for speech. So it is with every basic need. In order for a genetically determined potentiality or drive to develop, it must be animated by the appropriate stimulation, and that is by being spoken to or hearing spoken meaningful language. It takes well over a year to learn to speak, and we will speak exactly in the manner in which we have been spoken to.[13]

It is during the first year after birth that baby and mother most need each other. The baby needs to be held in her arms closely and often, spoken to softly, and nursed at the breast, to hear the reassuring, the continuing sound of her heartbeat. The newborn is a world away from her womb, but the physical distance is only a few inches, and the psychological distance is even less than that.

The mother needs the baby, too. All the time she has been carrying him, her body has been gradually and elaborately preparing itself for the role that it is now required to play, that is, to continue, on another level, the close relationship with her baby that was maintained during pregnancy. The enormous benefits that accrue to mother and child in this continued interrelationship cannot be overestimated, as it sets the pattern for a progressive development throughout the life of child and parent.

To sum it all up, it is through the love of the mother or caregiver that the child grows to be a healthy, loving human being. In the absence of that love the child will either wither away until it dies, or if it survives, not having been adequately loved nor having learned to love, will become "a cold fish" whose frustrated expectation of love leads to forms of disharmonious behavior, especially aggression, in one form or another.

Beyond all else, what we as human beings want and what we live for is the warmth and love of others, for love is the secret name of all the virtues.

Chapter Ten

Genes, Environment And Personality Development

*I*n the light of present-day psychological theory Joseph Merrick constitutes an intriguing case history. There exists a great body of evidence, both observational and experimental, which indicates that maternal love or its equivalent is fundamentally important for the subsequent healthy development of the personality. On the whole, this generalization appears to be sound.

Exceptions are sometimes encountered.[14] It is such exceptions that are often most illuminating, not alone testing the generalization, but also often extending our understanding of the variability of the workings of human nature.

And what is human nature? Is human nature something with which we are born, or is it something we learn? The answer to that question is not simple, but however that may be, the best we can do is to say that human nature represents the expression of the interaction between our genetic potentials, the environmental challenges to which we are exposed, and the third factor – which is usually overlooked – the developing individual himself.

Does the case of Joseph Merrick, "the Elephant Man," constitute an exception to the rule that maternal love or its equivalent during the first half dozen years of life is fundamental to the development of mental health? Without claiming too much, we have already described mental health as that attribute or complex of attributes, so varyingly present in human beings, which is characterized by the ability to love, to work, to play, and to think soundly.

Merrick's pitiable suffering in unrelieved anguish from his ever-worsening physical deformities made his life a burden of pain. Added to this hardly supportable load of affliction was, with few exceptions, the constant humiliation and frustration to which he was subjected by the world in which he lived. That he should have emerged from this unending rack of pain and torment so amiable and sensitive a spirit greatly enlarges, I think, our understanding of the nature of human nature. The deformed experience of Merrick did not lead to the development of a deformed personality.

Comparing the personalities
of Merrick and Pope, the poet

Alexander Pope (1688-1744), among the most gifted and accomplished poets, who from childhood was sickly, twisted, hunchbacked, dwarfed, aware during the greater part of his life that his deformities were the subject of laughter, ridicule and sheer cruel malignity, responded somewhat differently to his lot, even though he enjoyed so many greater advantages than Joseph Merrick.

No one could have been more sensitive to the ugliness of his misshapen body than Pope. He likened himself to a spider, a not inept description, for Pope lived in a sort of convoluted web of his own spinning in which it was his delight to entangle his victims, and pour over them his acidulous words so that they could escape not even from the passage of Time itself. The corrosive effect of his preoccupation with his deformities was evident to all who came in contact with him; it bit deep into his character, and by attrition gradually wore his integrity away.

As J. H. Plumb has written:

> All understanding of Pope must begin with his defor-
> mity, an ugly, terrible sight which he, as much as his
> friends, wished to ignore but could not. Like an ineradi-
> cable dye it stained all thought, all feeling. Deformity is
> commonly hideous in its effects. It corrodes character,
> leading to deceit, treachery, malignity and false living; and
> as often as not vitiates those entangled in the sufferer's life
> as much as the sufferer himself. So it was with Pope.[15]

But so it was not with Joseph Merrick.

Pope all through his childhood and youth received a good deal of attention from his parents, and was greatly admired by his early teachers, for from the age of 12 he was entirely self-taught, a Catholic in a Protestant world. He was early recognized and esteemed as a prodigy. Throughout his childhood he enjoyed the comforts and encouragements of a comfortable middle-class home in the country. In fact, Pope remained a pampered child all the days of his life.

In spite of detractors and enemies, the world of fashion, men and women of the highest station, the most distinguished writers of the day sought him out and lavished their praises upon him. Pope's writings had brought him considerable wealth. Yet he felt it necessary to pillory his detractors in such poems as *The Dunciad*: "The malice of my calumniators equals their stupidity. I forgive the first, pity the second, and despise both."

His words were brooded over and barbed, revealing the deep wounds that brought them forth. In spite of all the adulation, the slightest reference, intended or imagined, to his deformity would plunge Pope into an abyss of despair. From this he would emerge in frustration and rage, plotting eternal damnation and destruction of the enemy. He never managed to come to terms with his deformity. He could not live with himself. Nor could he live with others. In *Eloisa to Abelard* (1717) he acknowledged his own tragic fate:

> *Hearts so touch'd, so pierced, so lost as mine.*
> *E're such a soul regain its peaceful state,*
> *How often must it love, how often hate!*
> *How often hope, despair, resent, regret,*
> *Conceal, disdain – do all things but forget.*

In his vanity, malevolence, lying, doubledealing, rage, and contempt for others, Pope was clearly reacting to the ineradicable and intolerable image of his physical being, which had become so disastrously fixed in his own mind.

"There were few gestures in his life," writes Chard Powers Smith, "that were directed otherwise than to elevate himself or to debase a rival, and he was continually involved in one or more intrigues whose aim was to create the fictitious public figure not only of Pope the great poet, but of Pope the strong and courageous, the righteous and moral man. Somebody – I think Swift – said that Pope could not drink tea without a stratagem." [16]

How is it that with all the advantages of abiding parents, admiring elders, a country home, considerable wealth, the adulation of the fashionable and literary world, and above all the consciousness of his genius, Pope should have developed into so unpleasant a character, while poor, terribly more hideously deformed Joseph Merrick, whose mother died when he was a child, maltreated by a step-mother and an insensitive father, the victim of an unending course of the most brutal and painful experiences, should have turned out to be so amiable a personality?

The role of genetics
in personality development

One possible answer to the question of Merrick's personality is the genetic one. It is conceivable that the genes that may play a part in the formation of "temperament" or "character" were largely responsible for the differences seen in the behavior of Pope and Merrick. This is a possibility, but it is what Aristotle would have called an improbable possibility. There can be little question that genes play a role in influencing the development of temperament or character or personality, and that whatever the experiences with which those genes have undergone interaction, they have played a role in contributing to the structure of personality. That, however, is a very different thing from saying that the genes have played the dominant or the largest role in determining personality.

In the first place, genes determine virtually nothing. What genes do is to *influence* the physiological development and expression of traits. The manner in which that influence will operate will depend to a great extent upon the interaction between those genes and the environments or experiences to which they have been exposed. Genes without environmental stimulation remain inert.

Genetically identical plants when grown in the valleys look entirely different from those grown near the timber line. Identical twins separated from one another at birth and brought up in different social and educational environments may differ in both physical and intellectual growth in accordance with the differences in the environments in which they have been conditioned.[17] Yet genetically they remain for the most part identical. The power of the environment is very great, and differences in nutrition and education may make the most substantial kinds of differences in both physical and mental development.[18] As John Adams wrote to his wife, Abigail, "Education made a greater difference between man and man than nature has made between man and brute."[19]

It is not, however, the difference in knowledge or in social competencies that concerns us here, but the difference in temperament, in personality.

By temperament is meant the habitual frame of mind of the person. By personality is meant, in Gordon Allport's words, "the dynamic organization within the individual of those psychophysical systems that determine his unique adjustment to the environment."[20] In short, personality is the pattern of motivation and of temperamental emotional traits of the individual. It will be perceived that the terms "temperament" and "personality" have so much in common that they may be used interchangeably as having much, if not exactly, the same meaning.

In short, it cannot be said that Merrick was temperamentally the man he was because of his genes. But the matter does not end here.

Hereditary and environmental influences

Genes do not organize psychophysical systems, but environments, the social experience, the social stimulation to which the individual is exposed, do tend strongly to organize the expression of the genetic potentials.

The individual learns his adjustments to the environment for the most part, if not entirely, through the process of socialization, that is, the process whereby the individual acquires sensitivity to social stimuli, especially the pressures and obligations of group life, and learns to get along with, and behave like, others in his group or culture.

In the case of Merrick it is probable that genes played some role in influencing him to respond in the long-suffering, gentle, dignified manner in which he did – that is, adaptively, successfully – to the misfortunes that were so mercilessly heaped upon him. It was, of course, not simply or even largely the effect of genes that was being expressed in his gentle personality. There can be no doubt that to an appreciable extent his personality was influenced by the early experiences which he had undergone, that there had been an interaction between those experiences and his genes. That must be taken as axiomatic; but it is not an unreasonable assumption, in the circumstances, that whatever the nature of his early socializing experiences, Merrick's genetic constitution disposed him to make temperate, low-keyed responses to the challenges with which he was confronted.

Merrick's case does face us squarely with the "heredity-environment problem." As customarily posed, this problem is an utterly spurious one, since it opposes and separates the unopposable and inseparable, falsely assuming heredity to be something that exists as an entity in itself altogether apart from environment. This is a fundamental error. Heredity is not an entity one inherits, but rather, heredity is the *expression* of something one inherits; it is *one's genetic potentialities in inter-action with the environment in which one's genes have developed.* The expression of that interaction between the genes and the environment constitutes one's heredity.[21]

Hence, Merrick's heredity, like Pope's, and like every human being's who has ever lived, was comprised of both his genes and the environments in which those genes underwent development.

We know so little about the genetics of behavior that it is difficult for us to say anything with certainty concerning the development of any behavioral trait. It does not, however, seem unreasonable to suppose that the genes which are organized by the environment to participate in the structure of behavioral traits are characterized by an even greater variability than the genes involved in the development of physical traits. Hence, it would be expected, other things being equal (which they seldom are), that genes in any way related to behavioral traits would vary considerably in different individuals. No two individuals, not even so-called identical twins, have ever been totally alike in their genes or are ever likely to be. Considerable variability is the rule within the genetic constitution of every member of the human species.

That genes played some role in producing some of the behavioral differences between Joseph Merrick and Alexander Pope is possible, but to what extent, it is impossible to say with any degree of security.

Accepting one's lot in life

From what we know of Merrick's history it would seem evident that as soon as he came to be able to reflect upon his condition, unutterably miserable as he felt about it, he understood that there was no remedy for it, and that he would somehow have to live with it.

To continue to live as a human being, in addition to continuing to drag so deformed and pain-wracked a body after him, constituted an ever-present challenge to him – not merely to survive, but to survive and live with dignity. It must have been a conscious decision, in which, possibly, the predisposing genes were a help, for without such a conscious decision Merrick would easily have fallen into the accidie and bitterness of an Alexander Pope. He accepted his physical deformities and the pain of his body as a fate from which there was no escape. His role in life as an exhibition freak he also came to terms with, for he was aware there was no escape from that either.

But his mind, his soul, he knew was in his own keeping, and with the limited resources that were at his disposal, no matter how mistreated by others, no matter what the menace of the years, he resolved to remain the master of that one holy kingdom left to him. There he could live in imagination as he would.

In a way it was easier for him to live so than it was for Pope. Merrick knew that he had no more to expect from life than the lot to which he had been condemned – the possibility of any higher expectation, of relief from his disorder, of freedom to live as other men, was, he knew, beyond realization.   To that irrevocable sentence he accommodated himself. But with Pope the case was far different.

The more successful Pope grew the more this fed his awareness of the contrast between what he was and what he might have been. That the greatest poet of his day should have been, in his own eyes, the meanest man of his time, a misshapen, ugly dwarf, was a thought that grew with the growth of his fame, like an intolerable excrescence upon his spirit. The thought never left him and always oppressed him, his unsightliness making him unsightly to himself – indeed, sicklied o'er with the pale cast of thought – and exacerbated to the point where, accepted by everyone, he grew to be both unacceptable and unendurable to himself.

Critical developmental periods
and the maternal deprivation syndrome

Many of the traits exhibited by Alexander Pope are characteristic of the individual who as a child was inadequately loved. While Pope's parents may have doted on him in his later childhood, it is quite probable that they did not give him all the attention he needed during his first three years.

In the Western World it is the nuclear family unit, consisting of mother, father and children, that is the prevailing institutional influence in the socialization of the child, and in this unit it is the mother who is most closely involved with the child from birth onwards. So that for most children in the Western World the mother has been the principal agent of socialization, the chief molder, of the child.

It is one of the best substantiated hypotheses of modern behavioral science that in such families early experiences of deprivation will produce more or less serious and enduring personality disturbances.[22] And the earlier the deprivation of mother-love the greater is the damage done.

For healthy behavioral growth and development it is necessary for the infant to be exposed to the organizing influences of a loving human being. Under normally healthy conditions, the person best designed to serve as the organizer, the humanizer, is the biological mother.

There is now much evidence which indicates that there are critical developmental periods in the life of every child during which it must receive certain kinds of stimulation if its potentialities for behavioral response are to develop. These critical developmental periods are as follows:

1. The period during which the infant is in the process of establishing an explicit cooperative relationship with a clearly defined person – the mother. This commences at birth and is normally firmly established by five or six months of age.

2. The period during which the child needs the mother as an ever-present support and companion. This normally continues to about the end of the third year.

3. The period during which the child is in the process of becoming able to maintain a relationship with its mother during her absence. During the fourth and fifth years, under favorable conditions, such a relationship can be maintained for a few days or even a few weeks; after seven or eight years of age such a relationship can be maintained for longer periods, though not without some strain.

We find that three somewhat different experiences can produce the lack-love or maternal deprivation syndrome, and so interrupt a child's normal process of development. These experiences are:

1. Lack of any opportunity to develop attachment to a mother-figure during the first three years.

2. Maternal deprivation for a period varying for days within the first and second years, and weeks or months during the third and fourth years.

3. Changes from one mother-figure to another during the first four or five years.

Unless the child has been firmly grounded in the discipline of love and interdependency, he is damaged in his ability to develop clear and definite judgments concerning people and things, and his ability to form such judgments as an adult is seriously handicapped. As adults the judgments of such persons tend to be blurred and vague. Their decisions about the world, people and things tend to be characterized by doubt, suspicion, uncertainty, misgiving and unsureness. They vacillate, in short, they tend to see the world through a mist of unshed tears. They are characterized by an inability to enter into the feelings of others because, when they were young, no one cared enough to enter into theirs.

As mentioned earlier, it seems apparent that Alexander Pope failed to receive the love and attention he needed for healthy mental development during his first three years. On the other hand, Joseph Merrick's behavior strongly suggests that he had been much loved in his early years.

Put another way, if mother-love in the early years of the child's development is as effective in securing the development of a healthy personality as theory and observation suggest, then it is very likely that Merrick received a considerable amount of love from his mother during the significant early years of his life.

One can speculate on how this may have come about. By age three Merrick's deformities involved his head, his right arm and his feet. Though slight then, in comparison to what they were later to become, the pitiable state of the child must have elicited more than an ordinary amount of loving care from his mother. As his disorder progressed it is quite likely that he received increasingly more maternal attention, until her death, when he was not quite eleven years of age.

Chapter Eleven

Lessons Of
The Elephant Man

Man, in the unsearchable darkness,
knoweth one thing,
That as he is, so was he made.
                        –Robert Bridges
                        The Testament of Beauty

*I*t is, perhaps, more important to have told the story of
Joseph Merrick, the Elephant Man, than to inquire into
the conditions that made him what he was. No one who
reads this story can be anything but moved, even ennobled. As
he was, so was Joseph Merrick made.

But what were the influences that made him what he was?
There, some may say, lies the mystery. Mystery there will
always remain. It is difficult to circumnavigate the human soul
or even define it. It is, perhaps, more important to be able to
understand it than to define it. This we have attempted to do in
the preceding pages.

A sub-microscopic mutation in an hereditary particle, a gene,
caused Merrick to develop a disfiguringly hideous disorder
which would make him an outcast among men. Chance caused
him to he born into a poor family. Since he was already deformed as a child and grew increasingly more so, he might have
been abandoned at an early age. But he was not.

As we have seen, there seems to be good ground for believing
that he received much love from his mother during the first ten

years and nine months of his life. It was in large part this humanizing experience that provided him with the basic strength that enabled him to sustain himself and to surmount all the handicaps from which he suffered, to bear with courage and without complaint the martyrdom which was his lot every moment of the day.

This side of the grave Merrick had neither hope nor expectation of relief from the miserable conditions of his life. His situation was in every sense desperate, his physical agony exceeded only by his mental torment, a despised creature, a freak of nature, for whom there could be no consolation of any kind. To live with the reality of his physical hideousness, his incapacitating deformities, and the unremitting pain was more than trial enough, but to be exposed to the cruelly lacerating expressions of horror and revulsion by all who beheld him, was, we may suppose, even more difficult to bear. And yet, in order to survive, Merrick had to force himself to suffer these humiliations by exposing himself to the crowds who paid to gape and yawp at this monstrosity, the Elephant Man.

Never being able to venture out normally in the light of day, living the most ignominious existence, shifting from one manager and "impresario" to another, constantly on the move, badgered by the police, entirely alone in the world, knowing that there was to be no surcease, no amelioration of his condition, Merrick's hold on life, tenuous as it was, never weakened. His spirit remained invincible to the end.

He could, at any time, have cut the slender thread by which his life hung, but he chose to live. No matter what further bludgeonings Fate might have in store for him, Merrick was all the more resolved to go on. It were as if he had said to himself, "I suffer, therefore I am. And I am what I am because I suffer." It was, we believe, a conscious decision, at which he had arrived quite early in life, to live his life with the dignity of a man, to stand as erectly as he was able, and while the light from the pure flame that burned within him flickered, he would keep the faith with himself.

"Life is a pure flame, and we live by an invisible Sun within us." The words are from *Hydriotaphia* (1658) by Sir Thomas Browne (1605-1682) who, in another of his books, *Religio Medici* (1642), wrote the words which Joseph Merrick might well have uttered to himself: "Not that I am ashamed of the anatomy of my parts, or can accuse nature for playing the bungler in any part of me, whereby I might not call myself as wholesome a morsel for the worms as any."[23] But unlike Sir Thomas Browne, Joseph Merrick did not count the world a hospital to die in, but a wretched rack upon which the imprisoned human spirit, however tormented, whatever the mortal coils that hemmed it in, seeks unconquerably to express itself.

As Merrick is believed to have written,

> 'Tis true my form is something odd,
> But blaming me is blaming God;
> Could I create myself anew
> I would not fail in pleasing you.
>
> If I could reach from pole to pole
> Or grasp the ocean with a span,
> I would be measured by the soul;
> The mind's the standard of the man.*

One of the things we may learn concerning the nature of human nature from the story of Joseph Merrick is that given the adequate material to work on – that is, the genetic potentials – the love that the child receives during its first six years is fundamental for its subsequent healthy mental development. There can be little doubt that Merrick would not have come through as well as he did without the love he undoubtedly received from his mother.

Making every allowance for the genes upon which his experience had to work, we would nonetheless maintain that the love that Merrick probably received from his mother as a child constituted the principal influence in enabling him to respond to

---

*I have not been able to verify whether these stanzas were actually put together by Merrick. The second stanza is somewhat modified from a poem by Isaac Watts, "False Greatness," in his *Horae Lyricae*. (London, 1706, and many later editions.)

the challenges of his troubled life as successfully, even triumphantly, as he did.

In the love he received from his mother Merrick may well have had the advantage over Alexander Pope. Pope's deformities were as nothing compared with those from which Merrick suffered. His success as a renowned poet, his wit and wealth enabled him to live in comfort and move in whatever circles he chose. There could hardly have been a greater contrast in the conditions in which each of these men lived. And yet, Pope, as a human being, was virtually destroyed by his preoccupation with his physical infirmities, while Merrick managed to live with his far greater handicaps without being corroded by them. The genes that enabled Pope to become a great poet were insufficient to enable him to become a great man, to rise above his physical infirmities and proceed with the business of life, to be kind, to be, to do, and to depart gracefully.

But, as we have argued, perhaps it is this very contrast between the conditions of their lives that made it easier for Merrick to make the pact with himself that nothing more in this world could hurt him, and that he would make the best of his lot as well as he knew how. The contrast between his own physical condition and the conditions of his everyday life was all of a piece and nowhere nearly as marked as in the case of Pope. Contrast emphasizes difference, and the difference between what Pope knew himself to be physically and what he was as a poet, man of genius, and indeed the foremost poet, the most sought-after literary lion of his day, was something with which he perhaps could never come to terms.

There have been other writers who have suffered from physical handicaps. Remy de Gourmont, the influential French writer and critic, suffered from a disfiguring facial skin disorder. So did Sinclair Lewis. Remy de Gourmont solved his problem by seldom leaving his chambers. Sinclair Lewis attempted to deal with his with irascibility and alcohol. Toulouse-Lautrec, who was a dwarf, embarked upon a life of systematic self-destruction.

It seems to be the case that men of great gifts generally find the contrast between their physical handicaps and their social acclaim unmanageably difficult to handle. In this sense Joseph Merrick was lucky, in that there was little contrast between his physical handicaps and the conditions of his daily life.

Following his rescue by Treves, the contrast between his former way of life and the life he was enjoying in his hospital apartment could contribute only to Merrick's sense of near ecstasy. "I am happy every hour of the day" is how he put it. And all those who had a part in the making of Treves himself must have been happy, too: the shades of William Barnes, Thomas Hardy, Treves' parents and some of his mentors.

What is the moral of this story, if it has one? It is that the influence of a really good person lives on in the benefits he or she confers upon others, that that influence never really fades, and that courage and integrity are among the supreme virtues of humanity, outlasting even death itself.

On Our Reactions
To The Disabled

hy is it, in the Western World, so many people tend to react to the disabled, the handicapped, the "freaks" the way they customarily do?

These very terms, especially "handicapped," indicate an insensitivity toward those who are different, and different in what we regard as disconcerting ways — disconcerting to ourselves, that is. We are embarrassed by a confusion of feelings, and since most of us suffer from unresolved feelings concerning our own problems, we are particularly disturbed when we are confronted by those who trigger such conflicts in us.

These people are the innocent victims of a capricious fate. Their deformities remind us of the crippled image we are reluctant to face, of ourselves, an image we reject, from which, indeed, we recoil. It is the image we project upon these hapless sufferers who we think of as monstrous. But it is we who are the monsters, we who have become grotesque and misshapen, handicapped and disabled, because, among other things, we have become delinquent in understanding and compassion for the casualties of nature. It is the "freak," the "monster," who in a profound sense is truly the least monstrous among us.

Without thought or feeling we speak of "the handicapped," without realizing that in so doing we seriously handicap the innocent victims of fortuity.

There has been some improvement since the dark days when we spoke of the deranged, "madhouses," "insane asylums," or "hospitals for incurables," or exhibited human beings with deformities or disorders for the crowds to gape at. Children who were formerly referred to as "retarded" are today called "exceptional." Though there has been some commendable progress, there are still too many people who clearly resent the presence of the disabled – not only because they are reminded of the crippled image they have of themselves, but also because they are gratuitously reminded of their own vulnerability. Another reason they resent the presence of the disabled is that it stirs up their feelings of guilt for failing those whose needs are so great.

It is rather obvious that many disabled people are badly in need of adjustments in their own attitudes toward their disabilities. The phrase often used is, "I hate it" or "I hate being this way." So, clearly, it is not only the so-called "normal" who are in need of re-education, but also many of the disabled. The disabled often feel hostile toward the "normal" for confronting them with their abnormality, for "making" them feel "different" and "inadequate."

The disabled make us feel uncomfortable because we fail to relate to them. This is because we have become so isolated and encapsulated and so preoccupied with our own discomfort and disillusionment that we cannot tolerate adding the pain of others to our own. We tend to avoid the suffering of others as an unwelcome intrusion and flee from it as if it were contagious. We don't want to get involved. At best, we are embarrassed and don't know what to do, and by our awkwardnesses we communicate to the other our ambiguities and confusions. And although in such situations we might wish that we were elsewhere, we feel so not because we are uninvolved, but because we *are* involved.

In a very real way, most of us are disabled, more or less. We are handicapped by, among other things, our failure to recognize the kind of human beings we are able to become. The tragedy for so many of us lies in the difference between what we were potentially capable of becoming and what we have been caused to become by our socializers and our dysfunctional society.

If we will understand this, and understand how we came to be this way, there is hope that we may yet be able to save ourselves from the destructive course upon which civilized man has so long been bent. So let us begin at the beginning.

The able-bodied are only too often unsound of mind in their attitudes toward, among other things, the disabled. In their reactive revulsion, fear and awkwardness, they compound the injuries the disabled have already suffered. It is often easier for the disabled to deal with their problems than it is to deal with the customary reactions toward them.

I am afraid that we must first become human beings ourselves before we are able to respond to other human beings, whatever their disabilities or handicaps, for every human being is worthy of respect and compassion.

The disabled, the freakish, the deformed, and the "retarded" are a problem for many. The unexpressed wish has often been that they would just go away. Their presence bothers us, so we avoid or ignore them. But it goes deeper than that. We live in a disabling society in which most of us have, to some extent, been disabled as human beings. Our society has for too long been destructively dehumanizing.[24] On the personal level our dehumanization produces a defense against painful or overwhelming emotion, resulting in a decrease in our sense of identity and in the perception of the humanness of others – together with discomforting doubts about our own.[25]

The freaks, the disabled, whether physically or behaviorally, tend to awaken the wounded image we have of ourselves, an image we are reluctant to acknowledge. This results in resentment toward the disabled, followed by an awkward guilt for feeling as we do toward them, and embarrassment over our ambivalence, ambiguity and confusion.

Recognition of this fact provides encouragement, for the world of the future belongs to those who will bring us greater understanding, and with it greater hope. This hope is already in the process of being realized on two most important levels: First, in the understanding of ourselves as human beings; and, second, in the understanding, prevention and treatment of mental and physical abnormalities. Indeed, science now holds the promise for reducing the frequency of virtually every kind of abnormality — and thus for making the pain and suffering that accompany disfiguring disorders a thing of the past.

The Autobiography Of Joseph Carey Merrick

The following essay was written by Joseph Merrick as a means of promoting his exhibition in circus side shows. His promoters published the story in a pamphlet which they titled *The Life and Adventures of Joseph Carey Merrick*. It was sub-titled *The Great Freak of Nature! Half a Man & Half an Elephant.*

I first saw the light on the 5th of August, 1860.* I was born in Lee Street, Wharf Street, Leicester. The deformity which I am now exhibiting was caused by my mother being frightened by an elephant.

My mother was going along the street when a procession of animals was passing by. There was a terrible crush of people to see them, and unfortunately she was pushed under the elephant's feet, which frightened her very much. This occurring during a time of pregnancy was the cause of my deformity.

The measurement round my head is 36 inches. There is a large substance of flesh at the back as large as a breakfast cup. The other part, in a manner of speaking, is like hills and valleys, all lumped together, while the face is such a sight that no one could describe it.

The right hand is almost the size and shape of an elephant's fore-leg, measuring 12 inches round the wrist and 5 inches round one of the fingers. The other hand and arm is no larger than that of a girl ten years of age, although it is well proportioned.

My feet and legs are covered with thick lumpy skin, also my body, like that of an elephant, and almost the same colour. In fact, no one would believe until they saw it that such a thing could exist. It was not perceived much at birth, but began to develop itself when at the age of 5 years.

I went to school like other children until I was about 11 or 12 years of age, when the greatest misfortune of my life occurred, namely, the death of my mother, peace to her. She was a good mother to me.

After she died my father broke up his home and went to lodgings. Unfortunately for me he married his landlady; henceforth I never had one moment's comfort, she having children of her own, and I

---

*This is an error; the correct year is 1862.

not being so handsome as they. Together with my deformity, she was the means of making my life a perfect misery.

Lame and deformed as I was, I ran, or rather walked, away from home two or three times. But suppose father had some spark of parental feeling left, so he induced me to return home again.

The best friend I had in those days was my father's brother, Mr. Merrick, hair dresser, Church Gate, Leicester.

When about 13 years old, nothing would satisfy my stepmother until she got me out to work. I obtained employment at Messrs Freeman's, Cigar Manufacturers, and worked there about two years, but my right hand got too heavy for making cigars, so I had to leave them.

I was sent about the town to see if I could procure work, but being lame and deformed no one would employ me. When I went home for my meals, my stepmother used to say I had not been to seek for work. I was taunted and sneered at so that I would not go home to my meals, and used to stay in the streets with an hungry belly rather than return for anything to eat. What few half-meals I did have, I was taunted with the remark, "That's more than you have earned."

Being unable to get employment, my father got me a pedlar's license to hawk the town. But being deformed, people would not come to the doors to buy my wares.

In consequence of my ill luck my life was again made a misery to me, so that I again ran away and went hawking on my own account. But my deformity had grown to such an extent, so that I could not move about the town without having a crowd of people gather round me.

I then went into the infirmary at Leicester, where I remained for two or three years, when I had to undergo an operation on my face, having three or four ounces of flesh cut away. So, thought I, I'll get my living by being exhibited about the country. Knowing Mr. Sam Torr, Gladstone Vaults, Wharf Street, Leicester, went in for novelties, I wrote to him. He came to see me and soon arranged matters, recommending me to Mr. Ellis, Bee-hive Inn, Nottingham, from whom I received the greatest kindness and attention.

In making my first appearance before the public, who have treated me well – in fact, I may say I am as comfortable now as I was uncomfortable before. I must now bid my kind readers adieu.

> *Was I so tall, could reach the pole,*
> *Or grasp the ocean with a span;*
> *I would be measured by the soul,*
> *The mind's the standard of the man.*

Mrs. Kendal's Account of Joseph Merrick

From her autobiography, *Dame Madge Kendal* (London: John Murray, 1933, pages 282-285.) A rather better account of Mrs. Kendal than she gives of herself is in T. Edgar Pemberton's *The Kendals* (London: C. Arthur Pearson, 1900).

My husband saw Merrick at the London Hospital and on coming home I asked him, as usual, whether he had enjoyed himself there seeing the doctors and patients.

"No," he replied. "I have not. I have seen the most fearful sight of my life."

"Don't tell me about it," I replied.

"The extraordinary thing," declared my husband, "is that out of the distorted frame came the most musical voice. "

It so affected him (my husband) he could hardly speak. When he recovered he told me that Mr. Cardew had said they would never allow Merrick to be in the hospital permanently, although he ought to be there, as it was not fit he should be seen in public.

"Wouldn't they let him remain in the hospital," I asked, "if the money were raised to pay for his keep?"

I did raise the money and no one knew anything about my association with the case until the money was obtained and Merrick was duly installed in two rooms, one furnished as a bed-sitting room and the other as a bathroom.

His burning ambition. . . was to go to the theatre. A pantomime was running at Drury Lane, but how so conspicuous a being as he was was to be got there, how he was to see the performance without attracting the notice of the audience and causing an unpleasant sensation was the problem.

I went to see Baroness Burdett-Coutts and asked her to let me have the use of her box for the purpose. The Baroness asked if I would be responsible for what might happen to any woman who might see Merrick. I assured her that such arrangements would be made, that no one would see him either going to or from the theatre or while he was in the box.

This undertaking was scrupulously carried out.

My husband and I always considered it a great privilege to be allowed to soothe his suffering. He was most appreciative of everything I had done for him and expressed his gratitude in several letters to me. After his death I returned them to the London Hospital that they might be preserved with other relics relating to him. Enquiries made when writing this account revealed, however, that these letters are no longer extant, but in the museum in which his skeleton now hangs there is preserved a beautiful model of a Gothic church which he made and presented to me and I thought should be preserved by the hospital.

At one time Merrick wrote to me that he would like to learn basket work, and when I arranged for him to be taught he sent me the first basket he ever made. His love for music I fostered by giving him one of the early gramophones which worked by hand and, as I could not go to see him, he asked me for several photographs, which I duly sent.

His Majesty King Edward went to see him and when, in after years, the late Sir William Treloar gave a Garden Fête at Chelsea at which I had a stall, His Majesty on shaking hands with me said, "I think, Mrs. Kendal, you must have given your best photographs to James [*sic*] Merrick."

Lady Dorothy Neville, who also heard of the case, was another whose sympathy was so awakened on his behalf that she offered him a cottage on her estate for some weeks, on condition that he did not leave it until after dark.

His Royal Highness, the late Duke of Cambridge, gave him a silver watch.

Victor Hugo, The Hunchback of Notre Dame, and Multiple Neurofibromatosis

The following article, "Quasimodo's Diagnosis," by Lawrence M. Solomon, M.D., F.R.C.P., is reprinted from the *Journal of the American Medical Association,* Vol. 204, pp. 190-191, 1968. The references have been omitted.

Quasimodo's Diagnosis

The French Romantic novelist, Victor Hugo, was fascinated by the macabre and peculiar; he was one of the few novelists of that time who reflected the earlier compassionate views expressed by Philippe Pinel for the mentally retarded and insane, yet he peopled his novels with the violent and the grotesque. Hugo's observations were often acute, and he imparted his sense of the bizarre by realistic descriptions and contrast:

> Take the most hideous, repulsive, complete physical deformity; place it where it will be most striking—at the lowest, meanest, most despised stage of the social edifice; light up that miserable creature from all sides with the sinister light of contrast; and then throw into him a soul, and put into that soul the purest feeling given to man.... The degraded creature will then transform before your eyes. The being that was small will become great; the being that was deformed will become beautiful.

It would be interesting to examine the human source material for these "hideous" creatures of Hugo, with particular attention paid to the character, Quasimodo, *Notre Dame de Paris.*

Victor's father, Joseph Sigisbert Hugo, general in the army of Joseph Bonaparte (Napoleon's brother), summoned his family to Spain in 1811. Victor was 9 years old at that time and very impressionable. At the *Collège des Nobles,* a school which young Victor was attending in Madrid, there was a deaf-mute, misshapen dwarf who served as a porter. This unfortunate creature, called Corcovito (the little humped one), apparently haunted the author's memory for years.

Later the twisted dwarf was to appear as the wild Han in *Han d'islande* (1820), as Habibrah, the wicked jester in the melodramatic novel, *Bug Jargal* (1826), as the pitiful hunchbacked court jester, Triboulet, in *Le roi s'amuse* (the basis for the libretto of

Giuseppi Verdi's opera, *Rigoletto*), and later as Gwynplaine, in *L'Homme qui rit* (1869). The character of the hunchback thus evolved in several works and reached its maturity in Quasimodo, the twisted bell ringer of Notre Dame. Hugo described Quasimodo as follows:

> . . . that tetrahedron nose, that horse-shoe mouth, that little left eye stubbled up with an eyebrow of carroty bristles, while the right was completely overwhelmed and buried by an enormous wen; those irregular teeth, jagged here and there like the battlements of a fortress; that horny lip, over which one of those teeth protruded like the tusk of an elephant; that forked chin; and above all the expression . . . indeed, it might be said that his whole person was but one grimace. His prodigious head was covered with red bristles; between his shoulders rose an enormous lump, which was counterbalanced by a protuberance in front; his thighs and legs were so strangely put together that they touched at no one point but the knees, and seen in front, resembled two sickles joined at the handles; his feet were immense, his hands monstrous; but with all this deformity there was a formidable air of strength, agility, and courage, constituting a singular exception to the external rule which ordains that force, as well as beauty, shall result from harmony. He looked like a giant who had been broken in pieces and ill soldered together.

At the time of the story's main sequence, Quasimodo was 20 years old, able to speak only with difficulty, and deaf.

We know nothing about Quasimodo's family background. He was found wrapped in a blanket on a wooden bed in the Church of Notre Dame (where one left unwanted children) at about 4 years of age. He was so small for his age when he was found, it was at first assumed he was a newly born infant. When first appearing before Claude Frollo, the priest who adopted him, he was already misshapen, with crooked legs and a massive egglike tumor over his right eye, occluding it.

After death, his skeleton was found: "The spine was crooked, the head depressed between the shoulders and one leg shorter than the other...."

What was wrong with Quasimodo? We know that young Hugo, though much given to melodrama, was a superb observer – his early novels are panoramas with finely painted detail. We also know that Hugo was familiar with a real hunchback; and it is assumed by many that Quasimodo's description resulted from the novelist's remembrance of a similarly afflicted hunchback. If so, what was the probable diagnosis of this poor crumbled creature, so ugly neither man nor woman would dare look at him?

Quasimodo's disease seems to have involved three systems: the skeletal system with gross deformities, the nervous system with deafness and mental retardation, and the skin with a tumor (or tumors). It is also significant that Quasimodo saw perfectly clearly with his unaffected eye and that he was quite strong and well adapted to his deformity. The diseases which could explain such a combination of symptoms may be divided into hereditary and nonhereditary. The nonhereditary diseases do not adequately explain either the child's thriving in the face of his abnormality or his cutaneous lesions. We must therefore conclude that Quasimodo had a hereditary condition. Of the hereditarily determined diseases, possibly the best diagnostic choice is multiple neurofibromatosis, first described by Tiselius in 1793.

Let us examine the evidence for Quasimodo's having had neurofibromatosis by comparing the bony, central nervous system, and cutaneous changes found in neurofibromatosis and those ascribed by Hugo to Quasimodo. Among the osseous manifestations of neurofibromatosis, the commonest include scoliosis; congenital bowing of the tibia, fibula, radius and ulna; and pseudoarthrosis of the legs. Crowe *et al* found such bone changes in 35 of the 203 patients studied. These authors also found overgrowth of bone, with enlargement of one limb, a common complication of neurofibromatosis.

Spade-like hands and acromegaloid features may also be seen in the disease. Quasimodo's skeletal description corresponds, at times strikingly, to the bony changes of neurofibromatosis. Quasimodo had a tumor (Hugo used the word *verrue*, which more accurately translates as "wart") growing from his forehead and pendulously occluding his right eye. Could this lesion have been a solitary local problem? A veruca vulgaris would not likely be present from the age of 4 years to the age of 20 and achieve such great size. Dermoid cysts do occur in the region of the orbit, but they are not pendulous. A neurofibroma (molluscum pendulum) representing a systemic disease seems a better choice.

His nose simply protruded from the face with its fine features missing. The chin was "forked." The mouth was in the shape of a "horseshoe," with horribly deformed teeth – one tusk-like. He had difficulty in talking. Was this lower facial deformity because of skeletal, central nervous system, or soft-tissue changes in the mouth? We are not given enough information to say with certainty, but such changes as macroteeth, jaw cysts, and soft-tissue hypertrophy are seen in neurofibromatosis.

Quasimodo was mentally retarded and deaf. These two complaints are also seen in neurofibromatosis.

From the evidence presented here, it is probable that Victor Hugo's Hunchback of Notre Dame was a man suffering from

neurofibromatosis, and may rightly be considered the literary ante-
cedent of another interesting character with neurofibromatosis, Sir
Frederick Treves' "Elephant Man." Hugo's description of the vis-
ible aspects of his subject's skin, skeleton, and central nervous
system correspond quite well to what was to be fully described 51
years later by von Recklinghausen as neurofibromatosis.

The Nature Of
'The Elephant Man's'
Disorder

What was the nature of the condition from which Joseph Merrick suffered? What was it that so disordered his bones, especially his skull and skin, as to make him one of the most unfortunate of human beings?

His skeleto-cutaneous affliction caused him, among other things, to develop a head so deformed that it was said to resemble an elephant's. This was something of an exaggeration. The resemblance was exceedingly remote, and yet, it was there. For the purpose of attracting the attention of those who would be willing to pay their pennies to gape at a man who looked like an elephant, "The Elephant Man" was as good a description as any. And so Joseph Merrick became "The Elephant Man." The name was a showman's choice, and in no way bears any relation to the disease known as elephantiasis.

Elephantiasis is a disease due to infection by a threadlike worm (*Wucheri malayi*) which is transmitted by mosquitoes. Multiplication of these parasites results in obstruction and inflammation of lymphatics and hypertrophy of the skin and subcutaneous tissue. It is rarely observed during the first 15 years of life, and affects mostly the legs and external genitalia. The bones are never involved. Fibrous tumors (papillomas) are absent, although ulcers, small tubercles, fissuring, and discoloration of the skin often occur. Recurrent chills and fever are common. Merrick's affliction was of a very different character.

Merrick, in fact, suffered not from a disease but from a disorder.[26] A disease is an acquired morbid change in any tissue of an organism or in an organism as a whole; it has a specific microorganismal source and has characteristic symptoms. A disorder, which may be either acquired or inborn, is a disturbance of structure or function or both due to a genetic defect or to a defect in the development of the embryo, or as the result of external causes such as chemical substances, injury or disease. Disease is limited to malfunctioning of the organism initiated and maintained by an infectious process. For example, tuberculosis is due to a bacillus. It is an infectious disease which may, after it has been cured, leave the individual with a disorder or malfunction of the hip. The malfunctioning hip would be due to a disease, but remains a disorder. Merrick's lameness originated in tuberculosis of the hip, a disease which terminated in a permanent disorder.

A large class of disorders have no relation to disease. These are the disorders of genetic or embryological origin due to some error in the mechanisms of genetic or embryological development. For example, bleeder's disease or hemophilia, is not a disease at all, but a disorder due to a gene deficiency on an X chromosome. Extremely short or almost absent upper extremities, the condition known as phocomelia, with which thousands of European children were born in the fifties, was due to the action of the drug thalidomide, which was administered to pregnant mothers during the organ-forming period of the embryo's development, between the fifth and the twelfth week. Phocomelia is clearly a disorder, not a disease.

Viruses, bacilli, parasites, and the like cause diseases, and may leave the affected individual with a disorder, but most disorders are not caused by such agents, but are brought about by internal or external physical agencies.

The disorder from which Merrick suffered affected both his bones and his skin. In 1884-85 Treves had no more idea of the cause of Merrick's disorder than any other of his contemporary colleagues, even though, in 1882, two years before Treves came upon the Elephant Man, the disorder had been made the subject of a monograph. This was written by the German physician Friedrich von Recklinghausen.[27] Whether Treves ever knew of von Recklinghausen's work we do not know. Had Treves been acquainted with it it is doubtful whether he would have recognized the disorder described by von Recklinghausen as the same as that from which Merrick suffered, for the latter's disorder was so extraordinarily extreme it would have been difficult to associate it with the "disease" described by the German physician.

Von Recklinghausen was not the first to describe the disorder,[28] but certainly he was the first to recognize it as a distinct clinical entity. He had no idea, and could not have had any idea in 1882, as to its cause, but since he was the first to distinguish it as a recognizable "disease" it came to be called eponymously after him. It has been perspicaciously remarked that when a disease is named after some author, it is very likely that we do not know much about it. Today, in the matter of the disorder from which Merrick suffered, the case is very different.

Today Merrick's disorder is known as multiple neurofibromatosis or simply as neurofibromatosis. Now that the nature of the disorder is understood the eponym von Recklinghausen has increasingly come to be dropped.

Apparently there was no history of anything in the slightest resembling Merrick's disorder among his relatives. In his 1885 presentation of Merrick's condition in the *Transactions of the Pathological Society of London,* Treves states, "there was no evidence of similar deformities in any of his relatives." In the account of Merrick's death in the *British Medical Journal,* 19 April 1890, it is repeated that "there was no family history of any similar malformation." Neurofibromatosis often has an hereditary basis, and is usually inherited as an autosomal dominant.[29] The disorder is generally transmitted from a parent, and as is to be expected in conditions resulting from a dominant gene, fifty percent of the children will be affected. The dominant neurofibromatosis gene is carried on one of the twenty-two pairs of chromosomes and is never carried on the sex chromosomes. An autosomal dominant gene is one that usually expresses itself in the individual who carries it on one of his non-sex chromosomes.

Neurofibromatosis belongs to a class of disorders known as the neurofibromatoses. Neurofibromatosis is only one of an estimated 3,000 or more disorders caused by flawed genes. Two genes have thus far been identified as causing neurofibromatosis. One is called NF-1, is situated on chromosome 17, and occurs with a frequency of one out of 3,500 births. The other, NF-2, is on chromosome 22 and occurs in one out of 50,000 births.

NF-1 is distinguishable from NF-2 by the appearance of six or more cafe-au-lait spots, usually on the arm, before the age of two, whereas in NF-2 such spots are usually not present but may develop after puberty. In most cases of NF-1 the symptoms are mild; tumors may develop on the face and body, eyes, ears, and bones. Some children may have learning problems, seizures and speech problems and may be hyperactive; others may have large heads.

NF-2 is characterized by tumors that grow on the auditory nerves, often resulting in hearing loss. Sometimes cataracts develop at an early age, and tumors may occur in the brain or spinal cord, or even in the iris of the eye.

A child with a parent with NF has a 50-50 chance of inheriting the NF gene and showing at least some signs of NF sooner or later. Since genes come in pairs the child also has a 50-50 chance of inheriting the NF gene's normal partner and thus remaining free of

NF. Fifty percent of NF cases occur as mutations, and can have the same variety of symptoms as a person who inherited it from an affected parent.

NF occurs in every ethnic group in the world, and it affects both sexes equally. The defective gene is never carried on the sex chromosomes.

It is, of course, not possible to be quite certain that Merrick's disorder was without some familial hereditary component. A thoroughgoing exploration of Merrick's family history would have been difficult to make and was not attempted. Treves had, apparently, been in touch with some of Merrick's relatives shortly after he had met Merrick, for there is that reference to them in his 1885 report. Again, in the 1890 account of Merrick's death in the *British Medical Journal*, which was almost certainly based on information supplied by Treves, it is stated that "according to his relatives" Merrick had reached the age of 27 at the time of his death. (He was, in fact, four months short of 29.) The information that there was no family history of the disorder which afflicted Merrick was undoubtedly obtained from these "relatives." We know that an uncle appeared and testified at the inquest held at the London Hospital on 15 April 1890. He stated that Merrick had been deformed from birth. But a writer in the *Illustrated Leicester Chronicle*, who appears to have had an intimate knowledge of the family, wrote that Merrick's relatives declared that he was born a perfect baby, and that, "It was when he was about a year and nine months old that the first abnormality began to make its appearance." We may reasonably assume that the family history obtained was as complete as it was possible for the relatives to supply.

If, then, Merrick's disorder was not hereditary, the fact that it was congenital – that the infant was born already manifesting some of the deformities which were to develop so horribly as he grew older – suggests that we must look elsewhere for cause.

The fact that the disorder may have been congenital immediately reduces the possibility that its cause was either viral, bacterial or parasitic in origin. It is highly improbable that Merrick's disorder originated from any such cause. Treves especially emphasizes the point that Merrick's general health, except for an unspecified heart condition and bronchitis, was fairly good. He exhibited no evidences of infection of any sort, with the possible exception of tuberculosis having produced the condition of his hip. If, then, his condition was due neither to a virus, a bacterium nor a parasite, it can only have been due to some genetic defect. Genetic disorders are of two principal kinds, those affecting chromosomes and those affecting genes.

Chromosomal disorders take the form of some abnormality or abnormalities of chromosomal replication, the result of which is a loss of or an addition to the number or parts of chromosomes, or an abnormal arrangement of the chromosomes. Such chromosomal aberrations are known to produce in the body maldevelopments of every kind, depending upon the parts of the body and the particular chromosomes involved. Chromosomal aberrations usually affect development during the organ-forming period of embryonic life, the period from the fifth to the end of the twelfth week of development. As a consequence of such chromosomally influenced disorder, the embryo or fetus is either aborted or born with more or less clearcut bodily and functional abnormalities. Ears may be misplaced, the nose malformed, the eyes may be set too close together or are too widely separated, or the maldeveloped nose may be placed above a single eye, limbs may be malformed or incompletely developed, and so on. Virtually every tissue and organ of the body may be affected.

Such maldevelopments, due to chromosomal aberrations, have almost always been completed by the time of birth, that is to say, the basic abnormalities are more or less fully expressed. In chromosomal aberrations the malformed organs do not usually, after birth, undergo any significant change of form. Since such change did occur in Merrick, it suggests that his disorder was due not to a chromosomal aberration but to a defective gene, and so it proved to be.

A mutation is a structural change in a gene, usually harmful, resulting in a transmissible hereditary modification in the development of a particular trait. There are three primary types of mutation: (1) point mutations which involve changes *within* the gene's molecular structure; (2) gene elimination or chromosomal deficiencies; and (3) chromosome breakage. Any one of these three types of mutation could have been responsible for Merrick's disorder. Research showed that it was a point mutation that was involved. Whatever type of mutation was involved, its effect was expressed in a faulty control of the growth of the cellular elements of the neural, skeletal and cutaneous organs of the body. Of the many varieties of cancer it is now believed that some, at least, are due to such a failure of cellular control. In some of these cancers a virus invading normal cells may produce the destructively anarchic multiplication of cells which may run wild throughout the body. In other forms of cancer the triggering mechanism may already be built into the defective genetic system. In this connection, it is not without interest to note that while neurofibromatosis is, on the whole, a benign disorder, its tumors undergo a cancerous transformation, most commonly in males, in from five to ten percent of cases.

Merrick's disfigurement from neurofibromatosis was by far the worst ever recorded. Most cases of the disorder are benign.

As a result of the publicity "The Elephant Man" has received in its various forms as books, plays, film, TV specials, and many articles, reviews, and newspaper reports of cases, the media have taken to referring to neurofibromatosis as "Elephant Man's Disease." This is most unfortunate because there is not the slightest resemblance between anyone affected by the condition and an elephant. Furthermore, neurofibromatosis is not a disease but a disorder which affects women as well as men.

The media misdesignation conveys a wholly false impression concerning the nature of the disorder, and because it stigmatizes the victims and victimizes us into believing something which is not true, and because it brings pain and suffering to those who are affected by the condition, the description of neurofibromatosis as "Elephant Man's Disease" should be discarded. The acronym NF is good enough.

Proteus Syndrome, Multiple Neurofibromatosis, Neurofibromatosis, and Von Recklinghausen's Disease

Proteus Syndrome, multiple neurofibromatosis, von Recklinghausen's Disease or neurofibromatosis, as we shall call it here, is a fairly common disorder, occurring in about one out of 3,500 individuals. Fifty percent of the individuals presenting the disorder are the victims of a fresh mutation arising spontaneously in them. The rate, indeed, at which spontaneous mutations for this disorder has been estimated to come into being in each generation is 1×10^{-4} per gamete (ovum or sperm)—that is, in one out of each 2,500 to 3,300 births.[30]

Neurofibromatosis occurs in many different ethnic groups and in both sexes. In 94 percent of the cases there is either a loss or an increase of pigmentation with *café au lait* spots, most commonly on the trunk, though they may occur on almost any other part of the body. Mental retardation occurs in about two to five percent of cases, and seizures in about three percent. In the more developed cases the disorder is characterized by the presence of multiple, freely hanging pedunculated tumors irregularly distributed over the skin, associated with similar tumors along the course of the deep and subcutaneous nerves. The multiple tumors are composed of fibrous or connective tissue cells and nerve fibers, and are therefore called neurofibromas – nerve fiber tumors. Neurofibromatosis simply means the tendency to develop tumors of fibrous and nervous tissues. In most cases of neurofibromatosis the bones are not affected; in Merrick's case, however, they were.

The neurofibroma is composed of a profuse proliferation of the cells of the delicate connective tissue between the nerve fibers of a nerve trunk (endoneurium), as well as of the cells of the connective tissue sheath surrounding each bundle of fibers in a peripheral nerve (perineurium), and possibly also the connective tissue cells of the sheath surrounding a peripheral nerve (epineurium). Also involved may be the large nucleated cells which normally line the inner surface of the neurolemma – the thin membrane spirally enwrapping the fatty (myelin) layers of nerve fibers and the motor portions (axons) of unmyelinated nerves. It is the wild proliferation in the skin of the cells derived from these neural tissues with many nerve fibers imbedded in their midst together with large numbers of connective tissue cells that produces the typical disorder of neurofibromatosis.

The primary lesion in the skin appears as an unencapsulated nodule – an irregular rounded lump – covered by pigmented epidermis. The tumors may be soft or firm and range in size from a few millimeters to diffuse growths which hang in folds from the face, neck, and shoulders, all the way down to the abdomen. In their undeveloped form, as noted, the tumors may be limited to a scattered half dozen or more *café au lait* spots, ranging from localized nodules distributed over a particular part of the body, as on the back or forearm, to innumerable nodules of varying sizes over the greater part of the body. Hypertrophy – an enlargement – may occur in bones and in parts of the intestinal tract; there may be rib fusion and absence of the patella. Neurofibromata may invade various organs, and there may be fibrosing of the alveolar cells of the lungs.

Even though it is disfiguring, neurofibromatosis is usually benign. In cases of spinal cord involvement or the development of a malignant and metastasizing tumor, death is the inevitable consequence.

The Proteus Syndrome

Merrick's disorder was so bizarre and extreme that nothing like it had previously been recorded. However, in recent years cases of neurofibromatosis have been described in persons suffering from similar disorders, usually accompanied by seizures and mental retardation. These cases have been noted as a special form of neurofibromatosis, and named the *Proteus Syndrome*. The disorder is apparently due to a mutation, for there is no family history associated with it.[31]

Merrick's Skin
and Bone Lesions

The illustrations showing Merrick's appearance (Figures 12 and 13) require few words. Figure 12 shows Merrick at the time when Treves first met him in November 1884. This illustration represents an engraving made from a photograph. It was published as part of Treves' report on Merrick in the *Transactions of the Pathological Society of London* in 1885. At the time the photos were made Merrick was 22 years and three months of age. As can be seen from this illustration, virtually every part of Merrick's body was affected by the disorder, with the exception of the left upper extremity and shoulder. The former was perfectly normal in every respect and remained so throughout his life. The skeletal elements forming the upper extremity were also perfectly normally formed.

Quite otherwise is the gross overgrowth and malformation of every part of the right upper extremity. In addition to the overgrowth of bone and soft tissue the greater apparent elongation of the arm was due to the extreme curvature of the spine to the right from which Merrick suffered, as may be seen in Figures 18 and 19.

Merrick's right hand was completely useless to him. The fingers were so deformed and the palm so overgrown with fibrous tissue and disordered elements of the subcutaneous tissues that it could at most have served only as a sort of anchor. For all practical purposes his left hand had to serve him for two. It was with this one left hand that Merrick wove his baskets and made his remarkable models.

All the bones of the right upper extremity were more or less affected by the disorder. The humerus was thickened, and at its jointure with the radius and ulna much deformed. The forearm bones showed the ulna to be badly affected while the radius (on the thumb side) was much less affected.

That the skin was involved wherever the underlying bones were also disordered presents an interesting and significant correlation. Sheathed (myelinated) and unsheathed (unmyelinated) nerves enter a bone along with the blood vessels that supply it. The nerve fibers can often be traced as far as the bone-forming cells. Wherever the connective tissue cells surrounding the nerve bundles, between the nerve fibers, and around the peripheral nerves (myelin sheaths) were pathologically affected the bone became disordered. It is this fact that presumably accounts for the close skeletal and skin association of the disorder that affected Merrick.

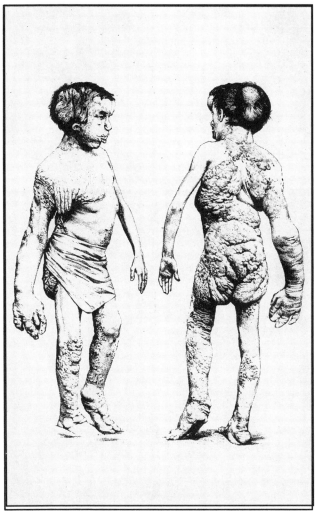

Figure 12. Merrick, as he appeared in 1884-85, shortly after being discovered by Sir Frederick Treves in a shop across the street from the London Hospital. These drawings from photographs are from *The Transactions of the Pathological Society of London,* Vol. 36, p. 494, 1885.

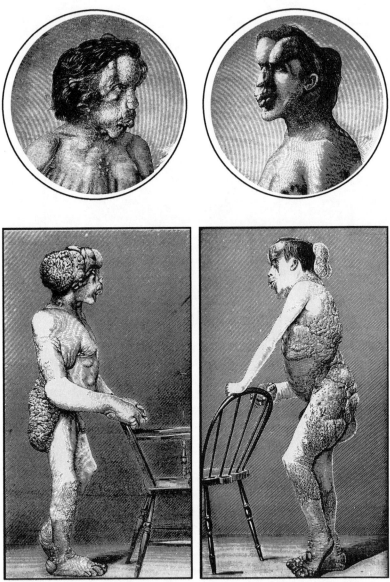

Figure 13. Joseph Merrick in 1886. These drawings from photographs are from *The British Medical Journal,* 11 December 1886, Vol. 2, pp. 1188-89.

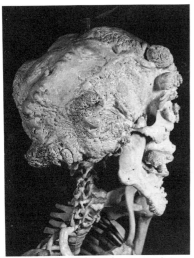

Figure 14. Right side view of the skull.

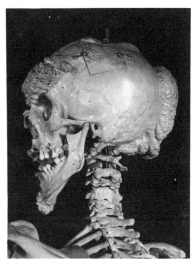

Figure 15. Left side view of the skull.

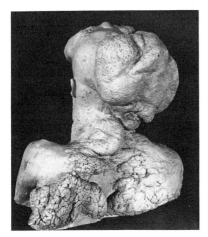

Figure 16. A cast, made after Merrick's death, of the back of the head, neck and shoulders.

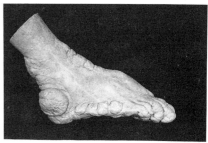

Figure 17. A cast of the right foot, outer view.

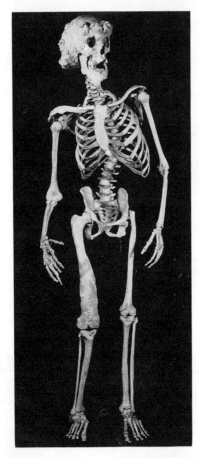 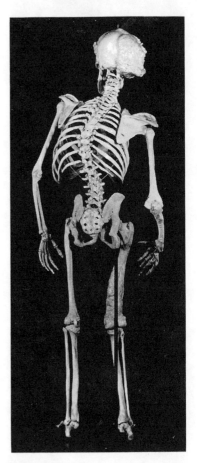

Figure 18. Merrick's skeleton, frontal view.

Figure 19. Merrick's skeleton, back view.

Returning to Merrick's appearance in 1884-85, as shown in Figure 12, we observe the massive bosses (elevations) on his forehead, due to the underlying enormous overgrowths of bone, and the growths at the back and side of his head, involving on the right side the ear, jaw and neck. Hanging from below his shoulder, on the right side, in front of his armpit, are several massive folds of skin. Opposite the fold on his right arm there is a growth of numerous tubercles. Both legs also show an extensive distribution of such tubercles. The feet are badly deformed and exhibit a considerable overgrowth of massive tubercles. The malformation and size of his feet required the sewing of specially made boots.

The apparent clubfoot on the left side was principally due to disease of the hip and thighbone. This caused Merrick to walk with a marked limp, and disabled him from standing for long without support. The diffuse lobulated tumors which covered the back and buttocks appear to have progressively worsened, as may be judged from the photographs made in 1886 (Figure 13). The papillomas which covered Merrick's body are branching or lobulated benign tumors derived from the layer of cells which covers the internal and external surfaces of the body, including vessels and cavities. Such cells are known as epithelial cells, and the tumors associated with them generally involve glands and related structures.

The odor which Treves mentions as emanating from Merrick's skin was undoubtedly derived from the secretions of the innumerable disordered sebaceous and sweat glands disseminated throughout these tumors. With the limited opportunities for bathing Merrick enjoyed prior to his rehabilitation, the accumulated bacterial decomposition of the secretions from the sweat and sebaceous glands would have given him a nauseating odor. This, too, must have added to Merrick's misery. The daily baths he was able to take following his settlement in his new hospital quarters completely eliminated this odor, thus indicating that it was in no way due to some abnormality of the sweat and sebaceous glands themselves.

The external genitalia, penis, scrotum and testes, appear to have been entirely normal and free of any form of disorder. This would independently tend to confirm Treves' statement that Merrick's "bodily deformity had left unmarred the instincts and feelings of his years. He was amorous. He would have liked to have been a lover." It was, alas, an experience Merrick was never to know.

A much clearer view of the tumors affecting the back and right side of the head, the back of the neck, and the back may be obtained from the photograph of the cast of these areas made immediately after his death (Figure 16). As may be seen from this closeup view, no area is actually free of involvement, with the exception of the upper part of the left shoulder and a small portion of the left scalp.

The delicately sculptured left ear remained almost completely uninvolved, though it seems to have been affected at the ear lobe, which was not free but attached to the side of the head. As the disorder progressed the right ear was rotated, deformed and almost completely engulfed by the enormous tumorous overgrowth. Hearing on the right side was probably considerably reduced, if it existed at all.

The only normal-appearing part of Merrick's head was a part of the left side of the scalp and left face from the upper eyelid, excluding the lips to the lower jaw. The unaffected part of the scalp was covered with a mass of brown hair. As would be expected, the only underlying bony elements on this left side of the head and face which were not affected were those entering into the formation of the "cheek-bone" (maxilla, zygomatic, zygomatic process of the temporal), the temporal bone, the great wing of the sphenoid, the squama of the temporal, the mastoid process, and the parts of the frontal and parietal bones above the squama.

This continued correlation of unaffected underlying bone with unaffected overlying cutaneous structures, together with the equally marked association of disordered underlying bone with disordered overlying integument, indicates strongly that the disorder spread along the course of the connective tissue cells of the nerve sheaths and those between and around the nerve fibers originating from the same main nerve trunks or branches.

The forehead, face and jaws of the right side were the result of the disorder spreading along the course of the ophthalmic, maxillary and mandibular divisions of the trigeminal (fifth) nerve and its branches. On the right side every part of the face is affected, including the upper and lower eyelids, the infraorbital region, the nose beyond the midline, the maxillary and the mandibular areas.

To the right of the midline of the lower jaw a great bony tumor grew from its body (Figure 14). This served to pull the overlying soft tissues and the lips toward the right. A tumorous growth from the right upper jaw and palate further served to deform the tooth-bearing portions of the upper and lower jaws, and since, as a consequence of these tumors, the jaws could not be properly closed, the vertical portion of the lower jaw on this right side especially has undergone considerable elongation and the molar teeth some displacement and rotation. On the left side the upper and lower jaws are unaffected by tumorous growths, but there has been some thinning of the bone and rotation of the molar teeth in the upper jaw.

Eating at best could not have been easy for Merrick, and chewing must always have remained a problem. And until they were removed surgically, the fibrous growths from his palate must seriously have interfered with his ability to masticate his food and to swallow. His teeth seem to have been singularly free of cavities.

Figures 18 and 19 show the front and back views of the complete skeleton. From these views it may be seen that the only normal bones in the whole body of Merrick were the bones of the left upper extremity, shoulder girdle and most of the ribs—all on the left side. The only bone on the right side which seems to have been unaffected is the shoulder blade (scapula) at the back.

The curvature (scoliosis) of the spine is markedly to the left. Almost all the vertebrae are to some extent affected by the disorder. The hip bones are quite misshapen. The right thigh bone is badly disordered and overgrown, especially in its lower two-thirds. On the left the thigh bone is thinned out and has lost its head to the disease of the hip joint in which the socket, wherein the head of the thigh bone normally lodges, is also virtually obliterated. It was disease of the left hip joint which was largely responsible for Merrick's disabling limp. The asymmetry and different lengths of the bones of the right and left lower limbs are evident from Figures 18 and 19.

Death of The Elephant Man

A report of the death of The Elephant Man in *The British Medical Journal,* 19 April 1890, pp. 916-917.

In December 1886, a series of drawings of this afflicted person appeared in the *Journal.* Since that date, the patient lived at the London Hospital. On Friday, April 11th, he died under circumstances which will presently be stated, having reached the age of 27, according to his relatives. His age must therefore have been overstated four years ago, as then he was believed to be 27.

He derived the name by which he was known from the proboscis-like projection of his nose and lips, together with the peculiar shape of his deformed forehead. His real name was Joseph Merrick. He was victimised by showmen for a time; when shown in the Whitechapel Road, the police stopped the exhibition. He was afterwards exhibited in Belgium, where he was plundered of his savings. On one occasion a steamboat captain refused to take him as a passenger.

The "Elephant Man" was twice exhibited before the Pathological Society by Mr. Treves. His complaint was not elephantiasis, but a complication of congenital hypertrophy of certain bones, with pachydermatocele and papilloma of the skin. He was born at Leicester, and there was no family history of any similar malformation. He gave an elaborate account of a shock experienced by his mother shortly before his birth, when knocked down by an elephant at a circus. It is almost certain that he was born with enlargement of the bones of the skull, right arm, and feet. When a child his skin was simply thickened, loose, and rough. He suffered in youth from disease of the left hip-joint, which caused permanent lameness. As he grew up, papillary masses developed on his skin, especially over the back, the buttocks, and the occiput. In the right pectoral region, the posterior aspect of the right axilla, and over the buttocks, the affected skin formed heavy pendulous flaps; a considerable part of the surface of the body, including the left arm, remained free from disease.

After his exhibition at the Pathological Society, the disease rapidly advanced. The fingers became crippled by hypertrophy of their integument. His general health remained good, and he possessed a fair amount of muscular power.

Such was the condition of the patient when last described in the *Journal*. He was then in a relatively flourishing condition, still able to go about. It remains for us to say a few words on poor Merrick's last days and death.

The bony masses and pendulous flaps of skin grew steadily. The outgrowth from the upper jaw and its integument – the so-called trunk – increased so as to render his speech more and more difficult to understand. The most serious feature, however, in the patient's illness was the increasing size of the head, which ultimately caused his death. The head grew so heavy that at length he had great difficulty in holding it up. He slept in a sitting or crouching position, with his hands clasped over his legs, and his head on his knees. If he lay down the heavy head tended to fall back and produce a sense of suffocation.

Nevertheless, the general health of the "Elephant Man" was relatively good shortly before his death. Early last week he was in excellent spirits, writing letters. He was out in the garden of the London Hospital on the night of April 10th. At 1:30 p.m. on Friday he was in bed (he seldom got up until the afternoon) and appeared to be perfectly well when the wardmaid brought him his dinner. Between 3 and 4 o'clock he was found dead in his bed.

Mr. Treves, to whom we are indebted for the above details, is of opinion that from the position in which the patient lay after death it would appear that the ponderous skull had fallen backwards and dislocated his neck.

An inquest was held by Mr. Wynne Baxter on the body of the "Elephant Man" on Tuesday last, April 15th, at the London Hospital. Mr. Ashe, house-surgeon, said he was called to the deceased at 3:30 p.m. on Friday, and found him dead. It was expected that he would die suddenly. There were no marks of violence, and the death was quite natural. The man had great overgrowth of skin and bone, but he did not complain of anything. Witness believed that the exact cause of death was asphyxia, the back of his head being greatly deformed, and while the patient was taking a natural sleep the weight of the head overcame him, and so suffocated him. The Coroner said the man had been sent round the shows as a curiosity, and when death took place it was decided as a matter of prudence to hold this inquest. Mr. Hodges, another house-surgeon, stated that on Friday last he went to visit the deceased, and found him lying across the bed, dead. He was in a ward specially set apart for him. Witness did not touch him. Nurse Ireland, of the Blizzard Ward, said the deceased was in her charge. She saw him on Friday morning, when he appeared in his usual health. His mid-day meal was taken in to him, but he did not touch it. The Coroner, in summing up, said there could be no doubt that death was quite in accordance with the theory put forward by the doctor. The jury accepted this view, and returned a verdict to the effect "that death was due to suffocation from the weight of the head pressing on the windpipe."

We understand that the Committee of the London Hospital refused not only to permit a necropsy on the body of the "Elephant Man," but also declined to allow his body to be preserved. Although the verdict explains the immediate cause of his death, there is a reason to believe that he was subject to cardiac disease of an uncertain nature; he was certainly troubled with bronchitis.

The circumstances under which the "Elephant Man" obtained the benefits of residence in the London Hospital were fully explained by Mr. Carr Gomm, chairman to the London Hospital, in a letter published in *The Times* on Wednesday. The poor fellow was grateful, intelligent, and interesting. The Princess of Wales and half the celebrities in London visited him. Ever since he entered the hospital the Princess forwarded to him yearly a Christmas card with an autograph message, whilst from time to time the Prince sent him game. Lady Dorothy Neville, Mrs. Kendal, Miss Lankester, and other ladies also showed him great kindness in a very practical manner.

References

1. Keith, Arthur. Frederick Treves. London: *Dictionary of National Biography*. Oxford University Press. 1937, pp. 856-858; *Plarr's Lives of the Fellows of the Royal College of Surgeons*. London: Simpkins, Marshall, 1930, vol. 2, p. 430.

2. Keith, Arthur. *An Autobiography*. London: Watts, 1950, p. 253.

3. Royal Archives, Windsor Castle, CC/42/52. See also Georgina Battiscombe, *Queen Alexandra*, Boston, Houghton Mifflin, 1969, pp. 245-246.

4. Clark-Kennedy, A.E. *The London*. London: Pitman Medical Publishing Co., 1963, 2 vols.

5. Montagu, Ashley. *The Reproductive Development of the Female*. PSG Publishing Co., Littleton, Mass., 1979.

6. Anonymous, "The Elephant Man," *Illustrated Leicester Chronicle*, 17 December 1930.

7. Hammond, John L., and Barbara. *The Bleak Age*. Baltimore: Penguin Books, 1947.

8. Howell, Michael, and Ford, Peter. *The True History of the Elephant Man*. New York: Schocken Books, 1980, p. 83.

9. Gould, George W., and Pyle, Walter L. "Maternal Impressions," in *Anomalies and Curiosities of Medicine*. New York: Julian Press, 1956, pp. 81-85; Montagu, Ashley. *Prenatal Influences*. Springfield, Ill. C. C. Thomas, 1962, pp. 169-216; Montagu, Ashley, *Life Before Birth*. 2nd ed. New York: New American Library, 1978; Montagu, Ashley, *Growing Young*. New York: McGraw-Hill, 1981.

10. Bowlby, John. *Maternal Care and Mental Health*. Geneva: World Health Organization, 1951; John Bowlby. *Attachment and Loss*. 3 vols. New York: Basic Books, 1969-1980; Various. *Deprivation of Maternal Care*. Geneva: World Health Organization, 1962; Casler, Lawrence. *Maternal Deprivation: A Critical Review of the Literature*. Monographs of the Society for Research in Child Development, 1961, vol. 26,

no. 2; Ashley Montagu. *The Direction of Human Development.* Rev. ed. New York: Harper & Bros., 1955; Ashley Montagu, *On Being Human.* Rev. ed. New York: Hawthorn Books, 1966.

11. Neumann, Erich, *The Great Goddess.* New York: Pantheon Books, 1955.

12. Chapin, H.D., "A Plea for Accurate Statistics in Infants Institutions." *Transactions of the American Pediatric Society.* vol. 27, 1915, p. 180; H.D. Chapin, "Are Institutions for Children Necessary?" *Journal of the American Medical Assn.* vol. 64, January 2, 1915.

13. Montagu, Ashley, *The Direction of Human Development.* 2nd ed. New York: Harper & Brothers, 1955; Ashley Montagu (editor), *The Practice of Love.* Prentice-Hall, 1975; Ashley Montagu, *Growing Young.* 2nd ed. Bergin & Garvey, Westport, Ct., 1989.

14. Ainsworth, Mary D. "The Effects of Maternal Deprivation: A Review of Findings and Controversy in the Context of Research and Strategy," in Various. *Deprivation of Maternal Care.* Geneva: World Health Organization, 1961, pp. 97-165; A.M. Clarke and A.D.B. Clarke (eds.), *Early Experience: Myth and Evidence.* New York: Free Press, 1976.

15. Plumb, J.H. "The Dwarf of Genius." *The Spectator* (London). 4 January 1957, p. 23.

16. Smith, Chard Powers. *Annals of the Poets.* New York: Scribner's, 1935, p. 484.

17. Montagu, Ashley. *Human Heredity.* 2nd ed.: New York: World Publishing Co., 1963.

18. Newman, Horatio H., Freeman, Frank N., and Holiznger, Karl J. *Twins: A Study of Heredity and Environment.* Chicago: University of Chicago Press, 1937; Newman, Horatio H. *Multiple Human Births.* New York: Doubleday, Doran & Co., 1940; Shields, James. *Monozygotic Twins.* New York: Oxford University Press, 1962; Koch, Helen C. *Twins and Twin Relations.* Chicago: University of Chicago Press, 1966; Scheinfeld, Amram. *Twins and Supertwins.* Philadelphia: Lippincott, 1967; Lewontin, R., Rose, S., and Kamin, L. *Not in Our Genes.* New York: Pantheon Books, 1984.

19. Smith, Page. *John Adams.* New York: Doubleday, 1962. vol. 1, p. 220.

20. Allport, Gordon. *Personality.* New York: Holt, 1937, p. 48.

21. Montagu. *Human Heredity.*

22. Newton, Grant and Levine, Seymour, eds. *Early Experience and Behavior.* Springfield, Illinois: C.C. Thomas, 1968.

23. Browne, Sir Thomas. *Religio Medici.* London: Andrew Crooke, 1642.

24. Montagu, Ashley and Matson, Floyd, *The Dehumanization of Man.* New York: McGraw-Hill, 1983.

25. Montagu, Ashley and Matson, Floyd, *The Human Connection.* New York: McGraw-Hill, 1979; Ashley Montagu, *The Humanization of Man.* New York: World Publishing Co., 1962.

26. Montagu, Ashley. "On the Distinction Between Disease and Disorder," *Journal of the American Medical Association.* vol. 197, 1962, p. 826.

27. Von Recklinghausen, Friedrich. *Ueber die Multiplen Fibroma der Haut und ihre Beziehung zu den multiplen Neuromen.* Berlin: A. Hirschwald, 1882.

28. Neurofibromatosis was probably first described by Johann Schiffner, "Sehr merkwürdige Abnormität der meisten Nervenparthien an einem Cretin, etc.," *Med. Jahrb. d. k. k. öesterr. Staates,* Bd. 4, 1817/18, pp. 77-90.

29. For a full account see Vincent M. Riccardi, John J. Mulvihill (editors), *Neurofibromatosis (von Recklinghausen Disease): Genetics, Cell Biology, and Biochemistry.* New York: Raven Press, 1981.

30. Crowe, F. W., Schull, W. J., and Neel, J. F. *Multiple Neurofibromatosis.* Springfield, Ill.: C.C. Thomas, 1956.

31. Tibbles, J.A.R. and Cohen, M.M., The Proteus Syndrome: The Elephant Man Diagnosed. *British Medical Journal,* vol. 293, 1986, pp. 683-685.

About the Author...

ASHLEY MONTAGU, internationally renowned anthropologist and social biologist, has spent a lifetime examining and exposing some of the most widely held myths concerning humankind.

Born 28 June, 1905 in London, he came to the United States in 1927 to begin graduate studies at Columbia University in New York. He taught anatomy and anthropology at New York University in the 1930s, received a PhD in anthropology in 1937 at Columbia, and was professor of anthropology and chairman of the Department of Anthropology at Rutgers University from 1949 to 1955. He also taught at Harvard, Princeton and the University of California at Santa Barbara.

In a prolific book-writing career that has spanned six decades, Montagu has ventured into the controversial areas of race, child-rearing and relations between the sexes. Against a solid background of scientific evidence, he has shown the theory of racial superiority to be fallacious, has dismantled the notion that man is naturally superior to woman, and has been emphatic about the tremendous importance of proper child-rearing, socially, biologically and psychologically.

The Natural Superiority of Women (1953), *The Elephant Man* (1971), *Touching* (1987), *Man's Most Dangerous Myth: The Fallacy of Race* (1971), and *The Human Connection* (1979) are among his best-known books. Others include *On Being Human* (1950), *Life Before Birth* (1964), *Immortality, Religion and Morals* (1971), *The Nature of Human Aggression* (1976), and *The American Way of Life* (1967).

Dr. Montagu was the principal officer responsible for drawing up the UNESCO Statement on Race, the director of the Department of Child Growth and Development at New York University, the director of the New Jersey Commission for Physical Health and Development, and one of the scientists who drew up the bill for the formation of the National Science Foundation.

Current Biography points out: "During the 1950s Montagu was perhaps the best-known anthropologist and one of the most popular university professors in the United States."